Leonard A. Jason
Steven B. Pokorny
Editors

Preventing Youth Access to Tobacco

Preventing Youth Access to Tobacco has been co-published simultaneously as *Journal of Prevention & Intervention in the Community*, Volume 24, Number 1 2002.

Pre-publication
REVIEWS,
COMMENTARIES,
EVALUATIONS . . .

"Explores cutting-edge issues in youth access research methodology. . . . Provides a thorough review of the tobacco control literature and detailed analysis of the methodological issues presented by community interventions to increase the effectiveness of tobacco control. . . . Challenges widespread assumptions about the dynamics of youth access programs and the requirements for long-term success."

John A. Gardiner, PhD, LLB
Consultant to the 2000 Surgeon General's Report Reducing Youth Access to Tobacco *and to the National Cancer Institute's evaluation of the ASSIST program*

More pre-publication
REVIEWS, COMMENTARIES, EVALUATIONS...

"BREAKS NEW GROUND in the effort to discourage teens from smoking. CONTAINS IMPORTANT NEW INFORMATION on the effects of laws that penalize youths for the possession of tobacco. The detailed description of model laws regarding the sale of tobacco will be helpful to any community that wants to protect its children. . . . Covers many topics of interest to public health workers concerned with tobacco and adolescents."

Joe DiFranza, MD
*Professor of Family Medicine
and Community Health,
Department of Family Medicine,
University of Massachusetts*

"AN ESSENTIAL RESOURCE for anyone interested in promoting policy change and increased retail sales enforcement. . . . One of the greatest strengths of this book is its careful attention to the complex and dynamic ways that individuals, families, schools, police, retailers, and the development of ordinances interact to prevent youth access to tobacco. The book also develops two useful tools for immediate use by community practitioners."

Scott P. Hays, PhD
*Research Scientist,
Center for Prevention Research
and Development,
University of Illionois
at Champaign-Urbana*

The Haworth Press, Inc.
New York

Preventing Youth Access to Tobacco

Preventing Youth Access to Tobacco has been co-published simultaneously as Journal of Prevention & Intervention in the Community, Volume 24, Number 1 2002.

DONATED By : J. Ferrari (Lisle resident)

Tel: (773) 325-4244
Fax: (773) 325-7888
E-mail: jferrari@depaul.edu

Journal of
Prevention & Intervention in the Community

Editor: Joseph R. Ferrari, PhD
Professor
Department of Psychology
DePaul University
2219 N. Kenmore Avenue
Chicago, IL 60614-3504

 The Haworth Press, Inc., 10 Alice Street, Binghamton, NY 13904-1580 USA

The *Journal of Prevention & Intervention in the Community*™ Monographic "Separates" (formerly the *Prevention in Human Services* series)*

Below is a list of "separates," which in serials librarianship means a special issue simultaneously published as a special journal issue or double-issue *and* as a "separate" hardbound monograph. (This is a format which we also call a "DocuSerial.")

"Separates" are published because specialized libraries or professionals may wish to purchase a specific thematic issue by itself in a format which can be separately cataloged and shelved, as opposed to purchasing the journal on an on-going basis. Faculty members may also more easily consider a "separate" for classroom adoption.

"Separates" are carefully classified separately with the major book jobbers so that the journal tie-in can be noted on new book order slips to avoid duplicate purchasing.

You may wish to visit Haworth's website at . . .

http://www.HaworthPress.com

. . . to search our online catalog for complete tables of contents of these separates and related publications.

You may also call 1-800-HAWORTH (outside US/Canada: 607-722-5857), or Fax 1-800-895-0582 (outside US/Canada: 607-771-0012), or e-mail at:

getinfo@haworthpressinc.com

Preventing Youth Access to Tobacco, edited by Leonard A. Jason, PhD, and Steven B. Pokorny, PhD (Vol. 24, No. 1, 2002). *"Explores cutting-edge issues in youth access research methodology. . . . Provides a thorough review of the tobacco control literature and detailed analysis of the methodological issues presented by community interventions to increase the effectiveness of tobacco control. . . . Challenges widespread assumptions about the dynamics of youth access programs and the requirements for long-term success." (John A. Gardiner, PhD, LLB, Consultant to the 2000 Surgeon General's Report* Reducing Youth Access to Tobacco *and to the National Cancer Institute's evaluation of the ASSIST program)*

The Transition from Welfare to Work: Processes, Challenges, and Outcomes, edited by Sharon Telleen, PhD, and Judith V. Sayad (Vol. 23, No. 1/2, 2002). *A comprehensive examination of the welfare-to-work initiatives surrounding the major reform of United States welfare legislation in 1996*

Prevention Issues for Women's Health in the New Millennium, edited by Wendee M. Wechsberg, PhD (Vol. 22, No. 2, 2001). *"Helpful to service providers as well as researchers . . . A USEFUL ANCILLARY TEXTBOOK for courses addressing women's health issues. Covers a wide range of health issues affecting women." (Sherry Deren, PhD, Director, Center for Drug Use and HIV Research, National Drug Research Institute, New York City)*

Workplace Safety: Individual Differences in Behavior, edited by Alice F. Stuhlmacher, PhD, and Douglas F. Cellar, PhD (Vol. 22, No. 1, 2001). Workplace Safety: Individual Differences in Behavior *examines safety behavior and outlines practical interventions to help increase safety awareness. Individual differences are relevant to a variety of settings, including the workplace, public spaces, and motor vehicles. This book takes a look at ways of defining and measuring safety as well as a variety of individual differences like gender, job knowledge, conscientiousness, self-efficacy, risk avoidance, and stress tolerance that are important in creating safety interventions and improving the selection and training of employees.* Workplace Safety *takes an incisive look at these issues with a unique focus on the way individual differences in people impact safety behavior in the real world.*

People with Disabilities: Empowerment and Community Action, edited by Christopher B. Keys, PhD, and Peter W. Dowrick, PhD (Vol. 21, No. 2, 2001). *"Timely and useful . . . provides valuable lessons and guidance for everyone involved in the disability movement. This book is a must-read for researchers and practitioners interested in disability rights issues!" (Karen M. Ward, EdD, Director, Center for Human Development; Associate Professor, University of Alaska, Anchorage)*

Family Systems/Family Therapy: Applications for Clinical Practice, edited by Joan D. Atwood, PhD (Vol. 21, No. 1, 2001). *Examines family therapy issues in the context of the larger systems of health, law, and education and suggests ways family therapists can effectively use an intersystems approach.*

HIV/AIDS Prevention: Current Issues in Community Practice, edited by Doreen D. Salina, PhD (Vol. 19, No. 1, 2000). *Helps researchers and psychologists explore specific methods of improving HIV/AIDS prevention research.*

Educating Students to Make-a-Difference: Community-Based Service Learning, edited by Joseph R. Ferrari, PhD, and Judith G. Chapman, PhD (Vol. 18, No. 1/2, 1999). *"There is something here for everyone interested in the social psychology of service-learning." (Frank Bernt, PhD, Associate Professor, St. Joseph's University)*

Program Implementation in Preventive Trials, edited by Joseph A. Durlak and Joseph R. Ferrari, PhD (Vol. 17, No. 2, 1998). *"Fills an important gap in preventive research. . . . Highlights an array of important questions related to implementation and demonstrates just how good community-based intervention programs can be when issues related to implementation are taken seriously." (Judy Primavera, PhD, Associate Professor of Psychology, Fairfield University, Fairfield, Connecticut)*

Preventing Drunk Driving, edited by Elsie R. Shore, PhD, and Joseph R. Ferrari, PhD (Vol. 17, No. 1, 1998). *"A must read for anyone interested in reducing the needless injuries and death caused by the drunk driver." (Terrance D. Schiavone, President, National Commission Against Drunk Driving, Washington, DC)*

Manhood Development in Urban African-American Communities, edited by Roderick J. Watts, PhD, and Robert J. Jagers (Vol. 16, No. 1/2, 1998). *"Watts and Jagers provide the much-needed foundational and baseline information and research that begins to philosophically and empirically validate the importance of understanding culture, oppression, and gender when working with males in urban African-American communities." (Paul Hill, Jr., MSW, LISW, ACSW, East End Neighborhood House, Cleveland, Ohio)*

Diversity Within the Homeless Population: Implications for Intervention, edited by Elizabeth M. Smith, PhD, and Joseph R. Ferrari, PhD (Vol. 15, No. 2, 1997). *"Examines why homelessness is increasing, as well as treatment options, case management techniques, and community intervention programs that can be used to prevent homelessness." (American Public Welfare Association)*

Education in Community Psychology: Models for Graduate and Undergraduate Programs, edited by Clifford R. O'Donnell, PhD, and Joseph R. Ferrari, PhD (Vol. 15, No. 1, 1997). *"An invaluable resource for students seeking graduate training in community psychology . . . [and will] also serve faculty who want to improve undergraduate teaching and graduate programs." (Marybeth Shinn, PhD, Professor of Psychology and Coordinator, Community Doctoral Program, New York University, New York, New York)*

Adolescent Health Care: Program Designs and Services, edited by John S. Wodarski, PhD, Marvin D. Feit, PhD, and Joseph R. Ferrari, PhD (Vol. 14, No. 1/2, 1997). *Devoted to helping practitioners address the problems of our adolescents through the use of preventive interventions based on sound empirical data.*

Preventing Illness Among People with Coronary Heart Disease, edited by John D. Piette, PhD, Robert M. Kaplan, PhD, and Joseph R. Ferrari, PhD (Vol. 13, No. 1/2, 1996). *"A useful contribution to the interaction of physical health, mental health, and the behavioral interventions for patients with CHD." (Public Health: The Journal of the Society of Public Health)*

Sexual Assault and Abuse: Sociocultural Context of Prevention, edited by Carolyn F. Swift, PhD* (Vol. 12, No. 2, 1995). *"Delivers a cornucopia for all who are concerned with the primary prevention of these damaging and degrading acts." (George J. McCall, PhD, Professor of Sociology and Public Administration, University of Missouri)*

International Approaches to Prevention in Mental Health and Human Services, edited by Robert E. Hess, PhD, and Wolfgang Stark* (Vol. 12, No. 1, 1995). *Increases knowledge of prevention strategies from around the world.*

Self-Help and Mutual Aid Groups: International and Multicultural Perspectives, edited by Francine Lavoie, PhD, Thomasina Borkman, PhD, and Benjamin Gidron* (Vol. 11, No. 1/2, 1995). *"A helpful orientation and overview, as well as useful data and methodological suggestions." (International Journal of Group Psychotherapy)*

Prevention and School Transitions, edited by Leonard A. Jason, PhD, Karen E. Danner, and Karen S. Kurasaki, MA* (Vol. 10, No. 2, 1994). *"A collection of studies by leading ecological and systems-oriented theorists in the area of school transitions, describing the stressors, personal resources available, and coping strategies among different groups of children and adolescents undergoing school transitions." (Reference & Research Book News)*

Religion and Prevention in Mental Health: Research, Vision, and Action, edited by Kenneth I. Pargament, PhD, Kenneth I. Maton, PhD, and Robert E. Hess, PhD* (Vol. 9, No. 2 & Vol. 10, No. 1, 1992). *"The authors provide an admirable framework for considering the important, yet often overlooked, differences in theological perspectives." (Family Relations)*

Families as Nurturing Systems: Support Across the Life Span, edited by Donald G. Unger, PhD, and Douglas R. Powell, PhD* (Vol. 9, No. 1, 1991). *"A useful book for anyone thinking about alternative ways of delivering a mental health service." (British Journal of Psychiatry)*

Ethical Implications of Primary Prevention, edited by Gloria B. Levin, PhD, and Edison J. Trickett, PhD* (Vol. 8, No. 2, 1991). *"A thoughtful and thought-provoking summary of ethical issues related to intervention programs and community research." (Betty Tableman, MPA, Director, Division. of Prevention Services and Demonstration Projects, Michigan Department of Mental Health, Lansing) Here is the first systematic and focused treatment of the ethical implications of primary prevention practice and research.*

Career Stress in Changing Times, edited by James Campbell Quick, PhD, MBA, Robert E. Hess, PhD, Jared Hermalin, PhD, and Jonathan D. Quick, MD* (Vol. 8, No. 1, 1990). *"A well-organized book. . . . It deals with planning a career and career changes and the stresses involved." (American Association of Psychiatric Administrators)*

Prevention in Community Mental Health Centers, edited by Robert E. Hess, PhD, and John Morgan, PhD* (Vol. 7, No. 2, 1990). *"A fascinating bird's-eye view of six significant programs of preventive care which have survived the rise and fall of preventive psychiatry in the U.S." (British Journal of Psychiatry)*

Protecting the Children: Strategies for Optimizing Emotional and Behavioral Development, edited by Raymond P. Lorion, PhD* (Vol. 7, No. 1, 1990). *"This is a masterfully conceptualized and edited volume presenting theory-driven, empirically based, developmentally oriented prevention." (Michael C. Roberts, PhD, Professor of Psychology, The University of Alabama)*

The National Mental Health Association: Eighty Years of Involvement in the Field of Prevention, edited by Robert E. Hess, PhD, and Jean DeLeon, PhD* (Vol. 6, No. 2, 1989). *"As a family life educator interested in both the history of the field, current efforts, and especially the evaluation of programs, I find this book quite interesting. I enjoyed reviewing it and believe that I will return to it many times. It is also a book I will recommend to students." (Family Relations)*

A Guide to Conducting Prevention Research in the Community: First Steps, by James G. Kelly, PhD, Nancy Dassoff, PhD, Ira Levin, PhD, Janice Schreckengost, MA, AB, Stephen P. Stelzner, PhD, and B. Eileen Altman, PhD* (Vol. 6, No. 1, 1989). *"An invaluable compendium for the prevention practitioner, as well as the researcher, laying out the essentials for developing effective prevention programs in the community. . . . This is a book which should be in the prevention practitioner's library, to read, re-read, and ponder." (The Community Psychologist)*

Prevention: Toward a Multidisciplinary Approach, edited by Leonard A. Jason, PhD, Robert D. Felner, PhD, John N. Moritsugu, PhD, and Robert E. Hess, PhD* (Vol. 5, No. 2, 1987). *"Will not only be of intellectual value to the professional but also to students in courses aimed at presenting a refreshingly comprehensive picture of the conceptual and practical relationships between community and prevention." (Seymour B. Sarason, Associate Professor of Psychology, Yale University)*

Prevention and Health: Directions for Policy and Practice, edited by Alfred H. Katz, PhD, Jared A. Hermalin, PhD, and Robert E. Hess, PhD* (Vol. 5, No. 1, 1987). *Read about the most current efforts being undertaken to promote better health.*

The Ecology of Prevention: Illustrating Mental Health Consultation, edited by James G. Kelly, PhD, and Robert E. Hess, PhD* (Vol. 4, No. 3/4, 1987). *"Will provide the consultant with a very useful framework and the student with an appreciation for the time and commitment necessary to bring about lasting changes of a preventive nature." (The Community Psychologist)*

Beyond the Individual: Environmental Approaches and Prevention, edited by Abraham Wandersman, PhD, and Robert E. Hess, PhD* (Vol. 4, No. 1/2, 1985). *"This excellent book has immediate appeal for those involved with environmental psychology . . . likely to be of great interest to those working in the areas of community psychology, planning, and design." (Australian Journal of Psychology)*

Prevention: The Michigan Experience, edited by Betty Tableman, MPA, and Robert E. Hess, PhD* (Vol. 3, No. 4, 1985). *An in-depth look at one state's outstanding prevention programs.*

Studies in Empowerment: Steps Toward Understanding and Action, edited by Julian Rappaport, Carolyn Swift, and Robert E. Hess, PhD* (Vol. 3, No. 2/3, 1984). *"Provides diverse applications of the empowerment model to the promotion of mental health and the prevention of mental illness." (Prevention Forum Newsline)*

Aging and Prevention: New Approaches for Preventing Health and Mental Health Problems in Older Adults, edited by Sharon P. Simson, Laura Wilson, Jared Hermalin, PhD, and Robert E. Hess, PhD* (Vol. 3, No. 1, 1983). *"Highly recommended for professionals and laymen interested in modern viewpoints and techniques for avoiding many physical and mental health problems of the elderly. Written by highly qualified contributors with extensive experience in their respective fields." (The Clinical Gerontologist)*

Strategies for Needs Assessment in Prevention, edited by Alex Zautra, Kenneth Bachrach, and Robert E. Hess, PhD* (Vol. 2, No. 4, 1983). *"An excellent survey on applied techniques for doing needs assessments. . . . It should be on the shelf of anyone involved in prevention." (Journal of Pediatric Psychology)*

Innovations in Prevention, edited by Robert E. Hess, PhD, and Jared Hermalin, PhD* (Vol. 2, No. 3, 1983). *An exciting book that provides invaluable insights on effective prevention programs.*

Rx Television: Enhancing the Preventive Impact of TV, edited by Joyce Sprafkin, Carolyn Swift, PhD, and Robert E. Hess, PhD* (Vol. 2, No. 1/2, 1983). *"The successful interventions reported in this volume make interesting reading on two grounds. First, they show quite clearly how powerful television can be in molding children. Second, they illustrate how this power can be used for good ends." (Contemporary Psychology)*

Early Intervention Programs for Infants, edited by Howard A. Moss, MD, Robert E. Hess, PhD, and Carolyn Swift, PhD* (Vol. 1, No. 4, 1982). *"A useful resource book for those child psychiatrists, paediatricians, and psychologists interested in early intervention and prevention." (The Royal College of Psychiatrists)*

Helping People to Help Themselves: Self-Help and Prevention, edited by Leonard D. Borman, PhD, Leslie E. Borck, PhD, Robert E. Hess, PhD, and Frank L. Pasquale* (Vol. 1, No. 3, 1982). *"A timely volume . . . a mine of information for interested clinicians, and should stimulate those wishing to do systematic research in the self-help area." (The Journal of Nervous and Mental Disease)*

Evaluation and Prevention in Human Services, edited by Jared Hermalin, PhD, and Jonathan A. Morell, PhD* (Vol. 1, No. 1/2, 1982). *Features methods and problems related to the evaluation of prevention programs.*

Preventing Youth Access to Tobacco

Leonard A. Jason
Steven B. Pokorny
Editors

Preventing Youth Access to Tobacco has been co-published simultaneously as *Journal of Prevention & Intervention in the Community*, Volume 24, Number 1 2002.

The Haworth Press, Inc.
New York • London • Oxford

3∂∂
.∂967
P944

Preventing Youth Access to Tobacco has been co-published simultaneously as *Journal of Prevention & Intervention in the Community*™, Volume 24, Number 1 2002.

The Haworth Press, Inc., 10 Alice Street, Binghamton, NY 13904-1580 USA

Cover design by Lora Wiggins

Library of Congress Cataloging-in-Publication Data

Preventing youth access to tobacco / Leonard A. Jason, Stephen B. Pokorny, editors.
    p. cm.
    "Co-published simultaneously as Journal of prevention & intervention in the community, volume 24, number 1, 2002."
    Includes bibliographical references and index.
    ISBN 0-7890-1962-0 (hard : alk. paper) – ISBN 0-7890-1963-9 (pbk : alk. paper)
    1. Youth–Tobacco use–Prevention. 2. Tobacco habit–Prevention. I. Jason, Leonard. II. Pokorny, Stephen B. III. Journal of prevention & intervention in the community.
HV5745 .P736 2002
362.29′67′0835–dc21
                                              2002010506

Indexing, Abstracting & Website/Internet Coverage

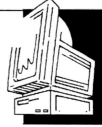

This section provides you with a list of major indexing & abstracting services. That is to say, each service began covering this periodical during the year noted in the right column. Most Websites which are listed below have indicated that they will either post, disseminate, compile, archive, cite or alert their own Website users with research-based content from this work. (This list is as current as the copyright date of this publication.)

(continued)

(continued)

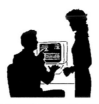

ABOUT THE EDITORS

Leonard A. Jason, PhD, is Director of the Center for Community Research and Professor of Psychology at DePaul University. He is a former President of the Division of Community Psychology of the American Psychological Association (APA) and a past editor of *The Community Psychologist*. He received the 1997 Distinguished Contributions to Theory and Research Award from the Society for Community Research and Action (Division 27 of the APA). Dr. Jason has published over 300 articles and 45 book chapters on preventive school-based interventions; the prevention of alcohol, tobacco, and other drug use; media interventions; program evaluation; and chronic fatigue syndrome. He has served on the editorial boards of ten psychological journals and has edited or written fourteen books. Dr. Jason has served on the review committees of the National Institute of Drug Abuse and the National Institute of Mental Health and has received over $16,000,000 in federal research grants. He has received three media awards from the APA and is frequently asked to comment on policy issues for numerous media outlets.

Steven B. Pokorny, PhD, is Project Director of the Youth Tobacco Access Project in the Center for Community Research at DePaul University. His research has focused on youth substance abuse prevention and public policies designed to prevent tobacco use among youth. Dr. Pokorny has authored and co-authored articles on issues related to media-based substance abuse prevention, self-governed substance abuse recovery homes, youth tobacco-control enforcement and crime rate, shaping youth access policy, future directions for preventing tobacco use among middle-school youth, and eliminating invalid self-report survey data. His formal training is in clinical psychology with an emphasis on community psychology. Dr. Pokorny plans to continue his research on community-level interventions to prevent tobacco use among youth and to utilize the findings to inform local, state, and federal tobacco-control policies.

Preventing Youth Access
to Tobacco

CONTENTS

Introduction:
Preventing Youth Access to Tobacco

Leonard A. Jason
Steven B. Pokorny

DePaul University

Carrie J. Curie

University of Kansas

Stephanie M. Townsend

University of Illinois at Chicago

SUMMARY. In this volume, we will examine different components of a preventive public health intervention directed at reducing rates of youth smoking. The rationale for this intervention is presented as well as a review of the literature on this topic. Five data-based papers will provide readers with an overview of different aspects of this large community-based preventive intervention. One paper will examine the types of ordinances that communities have adopted and what our recommendations are for optimal tobacco control policies at the local level. A second

---

Address correspondence to: Leonard A. Jason, PhD, DePaul University, Center for Community Research, 990 West Fullerton Avenue, Chicago, IL 60614.

The authors express appreciation for the financial support provided by the Robert Wood Johnson Foundation and David Altman, the National Program Director, and Andrea Williams, the Deputy Director, of the Substance Abuse Policy Research Program.

1

paper will examine the readiness of communities to begin the process of changing, and how that might be documented. Another domain we will investigate is whether the types of tobacco prevention programs in schools have an effect on youth smoking rates. We will also provide data about what influences a store merchant to actually illegally sell tobacco to minors. Finally, we will investigate whether youth who participate in tobacco purchase efforts become more likely to try smoking or whether their attitudes change as a function of participating in these programs. We conclude that effective programs are more likely to be comprehensive, sustainable, well planned, and coordinated at the local level. *[Article copies available for a fee from The Haworth Document Delivery Service: 1-800-HAWORTH. E-mail address: <getinfo@haworthpressinc.com> Website: <http://www.HaworthPress.com> © 2002 by The Haworth Press, Inc. All rights reserved.]*

KEYWORDS. Minors, tobacco, youth access, preventing smoking

Researchers have long grappled with the problem of reducing tobacco use as a way of optimizing the health and well-being of communities (Rhodes & Jason, 1988). From the early to the mid 1990s, current smoking, defined as having smoked in the past 30 days, increased from 27.8% to 34% for high school students, and increased from 15.5% to 21% for eighth graders (Johnston, 1996). Even though rates have begun to decrease 1 to 3 percentage points in the last few years, rates of smoking among American teens remain very high (Johnston, Bachman & O'Malley, 1998). Every day, 3,000 American adolescents begin smoking (Pierce, Fiore, Novotny, Hatziandreu, & Davis, 1989), and it is estimated that 1,000 of these children will eventually die of tobacco-related illnesses (Centers for Disease Control, 1996).

Smoking is the leading preventable cause of death in the United States, killing over 400,000 people each year. This is more people than die each year of acquired immune deficiency syndrome, homicide, suicide, automobile accidents, illegal drug use, and fires combined. The direct medical costs of treating tobacco related diseases in the United States are estimated at $50,000,000,000 per year (Centers for Disease Control, 1996). The amount of human pain and suffering caused by tobacco use is immeasurable. Despite these facts, 22.9% of adult Americans and 13.8% of Americans under the age of 18 smoke cigarettes (Centers for Disease Control, 1996).

The findings above strongly indicate that preventing youth smoking initiation is the most effective way to reduce long-term mortality from heart disease, cancer, chronic lung disease, and other tobacco-related disorders. There will always be some children and adolescents who use; the key question is whether there are behavioral and social data that indicate a way to reduce the number of children who begin this deadly habit. The most effective policies might be those that are universal interventions that both reduce youth access to tobacco products and promote tobacco-free norms through taxation of tobacco products, regulation of tobacco products, enforcement of youth access laws, constraints on advertising and promotion, and tobacco control advocacy for tobacco-free environments (Jason, Biglan & Katz, 1998). It is beyond the scope of this article to review all of these preventive policies, and below we will focus on the potential of curtailing youth access to tobacco.

ONE COMPONENT OF THE PROBLEM– EASY ACCESS TO TOBACCO

Nicotine addiction typically begins in adolescence with experimental cigarette smoking that progresses to smoking as a social activity and finally to regular, daily cigarette smoking. One of the risk factors for adolescent cigarette smoking is easy access to tobacco products (DiFranza, Carlson, & Caisse, 1992; Stanton, Mahalski, McGee, & Silva, 1993). In the US, research conducted in the 1980s up to the mid 1990s found that in most areas minors could purchase cigarettes from retailers most of the time (Jason, Ji, Anes, & Birkhead, 1991; Forster, Komro, & Wolfson, 1996). Findings also indicate that adults in the US overwhelmingly support policies that limit minors' access to tobacco (Strouse & Hall, 1994). Even though fewer vendors are selling minors cigarettes, due to recent legislative actions to be described below, youth still have easy access to tobacco products (Jason et al., 1999). There is some evidence that adolescents' attitudes toward anti-tobacco policies play a role in their decisions about smoking (Unger et al., 1999).

Educational programs have been implemented as a way to deter merchants from selling cigarettes to minors, but it seems that cigarette sales usually remain unchanged or rebound after time (Biglan et al., 1995). A study in California (Altman, Wheelis, McFarlane, Lee & Fortmann, 1999) found that intensive educational programs did effectively reduce illegal sales, but the communities were relatively small, and considerable educational efforts were needed to accomplish these results.

AN EFFECTIVE SOLUTION

In a study designed by the first author, approximately 70% of tobacco vendors in Woodridge, Illinois, were found to sell cigarettes to minors during a baseline condition (Jason et al., 1991). Community antismoking legislation was developed that involved licensing and enforcement. In the enforcement condition, minors went into the stores to make purchase attempts on a regular basis and police issued citations to merchants who sold cigarettes. Those merchants were also reported to the Woodridge mayor, who is the village liquor and tobacco commissioner. The mayor imposed fines and suspended the tobacco licenses of merchants who were found in an administrative hearing to have violated the age restrictions on tobacco sales (Jason et al., 1991). Minors were also fined for tobacco possession. After enforcement began, illegal cigarette sales to minors dropped to less than 5%. Student surveys conducted two years after passage of this legislation indicated that rates of regular smoking among seventh and eighth graders had been reduced from 16% to 5%.

Effective laws have several common characteristics. These characteristics are: (1) civil, not criminal penalties that are leveled against the store owner and not just against the clerk, (2) progressively increasing fees culminating in the suspension or revocation of a tobacco vendors license, and (3) regular enforcement of the law using minors in unannounced purchase attempts to monitor compliance. In addition, some communities have fined minors for tobacco possession. As mentioned above, the village of Woodridge, Illinois was the first documented case of a community that, using a law that had these characteristics, was able to reduce the sales rate of tobacco to minors (Jason et al., 1991). Feighery, Altman, and Shaffer (1991) found the combination of education plus enforcement reduced illegal sales of cigarettes, whereas education alone was not particularly effective. Studies have shown that reductions in youths' ability to purchase tobacco can be achieved through regular enforcement of these types of youth access to tobacco laws.

Efforts such as those described above are becoming common due to federal legislation. In 1996, the Department of Health and Human Services (HHS) finalized and published the Substance Abuse and Mental

Health Services Administration (SAMHSA) regulation implementing the Synar Amendment. The key requirements of the regulation require states to adopt laws prohibiting the sale of tobacco to any individual under the age of 18; enforce such laws in a manner that can reasonably be expected to reduce the extent to which tobacco products are available to minors; conduct annual random, unannounced inspections to ensure compliance with the law; develop a strategy and time frame for reducing illegal cigarette sales to less than 20%; and submit an annual report, detailing efforts to enforce the law, which describes how inspections were conducted, the methods of identifying tobacco outlets, and the overall success of the previous fiscal year to reduce minors' access to tobacco. In addition, the report must also include plans for enforcing the law. The Synar Amendment also requires the federal government to deduct 10% of substance abuse funds from states that do not comply with the regulations.

DO REDUCTIONS IN YOUTH ACCESS TO TOBACCO LEAD TO LOWER YOUTH SMOKING?

An important public health question arises of whether this reduction of minors' ability to purchase tobacco has any effect on the level of cigarette smoking among youth. In a study of 12- to 19-year-olds in Massachusetts conducted by DiFranza, Carlson, and Caisse (1992), two years after legislation was passed that enforced tobacco access laws, the percentage of students identifying themselves as smokers dropped from 22.8% to 15.8%. In another study conducted in Washington, within a year of the initiation of compliance checks, regular tobacco use fell from 22% to 14% for younger adolescents (i.e., ages 14 to 15 years old), whereas the rate rose from 31% to 35% for older students (i.e., ages 16 to 17 years old) (Hinds, 1992). Forster, Murray, Wolfson, Blaine, Wagenaar, and Hennrikus (1998) found a 4.9% reduction in daily smoking for youth in cities exposed to enforcement of a comprehensive youth access ordinance compared to control cities. In Woodridge, Illinois, the smoking rate among seventh and eighth graders decreased considerably after two years of enforcement using compliance checks and fining minors for tobacco possession (Jason et al., 1991). Seven-year follow-up data were collected in five towns; two had regular enforcement and fines for tobacco possession (Woodridge and a neighboring town) and three towns did not have regular enforcement. High school students who lived in communities with regular enforcement reported significantly less tobacco possession than those living in communities without regular enforcement (8.1% vs. 15.5%, respectively; Jason et al., 1999).

In contrast, a study by Rigotti et al. (1997) found that enforcement in three communities, when compared to three control communities, did not lead to reductions in youth tobacco use; however, self-reported access to tobacco remained at high levels in both experimental and control communities. In the Rigotti et al. (1997) study, it is possible that findings were affected by the absence of significant differences between the percentage of youth that purchased tobacco in the experimental as compared to the control conditions.

It is possible that some of the differences between the findings in Woodridge (Jason et al., 1999) and those of Rigotti et al. (1997) result from lower sales rates to minors and fining minors for tobacco possession. Rigotti et al. (1997) had intended to obtain merchant compliance of 90%, but they were only able to reach a compliance rate of 82% (baseline rates were 35%). Compliance checks occurred in an average of 0.5 per vendor in control communities, and this might have influenced the findings, as compliance in control communities increased from 28% to 45% over the two year study. In addition, student respondees were only sampled in high schools in the Rigotti et al. (1997) study, not in junior high schools, a time when decisions about smoking often occur. Finally, because even with strict enforcement, cigarettes are often still available, it might be important also to fine minors for tobacco possession in order to decrease the prevalence of smoking, as was done in Woodridge.

As Rigotti et al. (1997) mention, there are several ways of explaining their findings. Only one store might sell tobacco products to underage youth, and youth who smoke might only purchase cigarettes at that store. Some youth probably purchase cigarettes in neighboring towns or from older youth, but this might occur more often in high school as opposed to junior high school youth. Some youth might obtain cigarettes by using false identification, dressing to look older, and saying that they are over 18, but these behaviors might also occur more frequently in older rather than younger minors.

A study by Altman et al. (1999) compared two treatment communities with two control communities. Over a three year period, the treatment communities received a diverse array of community interventions, including community education, merchant education, and voluntary policy change. In the treatment communities, the percentage of stores selling to minors dropped from 75% at the baseline assessment to 0% at the final assessment; whereas in the control communities, rates dropped from 64% to 39%. When examining tobacco use in the past 30 days, 7th graders in the treatment communities were significantly less likely to use tobacco (rates lowered from 13.1% to 12.6%), whereas rates increased in the comparison communities (from 15.6% to 18.6%). Significant effects were not found in the 9th or 11th grades. The authors conclude that commercial sources of tobacco sales may have been influenced by the intervention, but students were still able to buy tobacco from other means (e.g., asking others to buy it for them, using fake IDs, and stealing).

These findings suggest that the effects of these types of programs on prevalence might be most evident among younger students, and since tobacco is still readily available to youth, more comprehensive programs (e.g., fining minors for tobacco possession) might need to be combined with efforts to restrict merchants from illegally selling tobacco products to minors. Economic theory (Chaloupka & Pacula, 1998) of supply and demand suggests that with merchants less likely to sell tobacco to youth, minors will increasingly rely on social sources to obtain their cigarettes. However, costs of obtaining cigarettes might be increased when both merchants do not sell tobacco to youth and minors are fined for possession of tobacco, and such a theory might be used to support the hypothesis that reductions in youth tobacco use are best achievable by actively enforcing both minimum age to purchase tobacco and youth possession laws.

There still is controversy about whether to fine minors for possession of cigarettes (Forster & Wolfson, 1998). Some anti-smoking coalitions, like Smoke-Free Pennsylvania, are opposed to these measures because they might make the youth the offender rather than the victim of the tobacco industry's efforts to recruit new smokers. By shifting enforcement efforts to teenagers, the real offenders who sell these deadly products are protected from being fined. While focusing just on fining youth for possession of tobacco is inappropriate, a combined approach involving both fining merchants for illegal sales of tobacco and youth for possession of tobacco is appropriate. Talbot (1992) believes that we need to focus both on fining merchants who sell tobacco products to minors and minors who possess tobacco products. Talbot argues that possession bans make it easier to reduce subtle peer pressure when students congregate at social events and publicly smoke and encourage others to engage in this behavior. There is a clear need to investigate this issue further and determine whether these policies might influence rates of smoking among youth.

ROBERT WOOD JOHNSON SUPPORTED RESEARCH: DEPAUL UNIVERSITY STUDIES

If merchants are less likely to sell tobacco to youth, minors might increasingly rely on social sources to obtain their cigarettes. However, costs of obtaining cigarettes might be increased only when both merchants do not sell tobacco to youth and minors are fined for possession of tobacco, and economic theory of supply and demand might be used to support the hypothesis that reductions in youth tobacco use are best achievable by actively enforcing both tobacco sales and youth possession laws. The Robert Wood Johnson supported study occurred from 1999 until 2001, and involved a randomized test of the hypothesis that the combination of enforcements plus fines would be more effective in reducing youth smoking than enforcements alone.

Sixty-eight towns, each with a population of at least 5,000, were initially contacted, and 26 met criteria (i.e., low levels of enforcement and fines for minors possessing tobacco) based on data provided during telephone conversations with officials at the police departments. Twenty-one police chiefs from these 26 communities agreed to be in the study, and each had to be willing to be randomized to two experimental conditions. Eleven of these 21 towns had superintendents and principals that agreed to be in the study. One of these towns was excluded because we learned that they were implementing high rates of sales enforcements and minor fines prior to the start of our study. The remaining ten towns were randomly assigned to one of two conditions: Possession (P) enforcement of both tobacco possession and sales laws, or No Possession (NP) enforcement of only the tobacco sales law. These towns were matched for population size and median family income before they were randomly assigned to the conditions. After more contact with the police departments, we later learned that two of these towns were fining minors for tobacco possession at a rate over .15% (number of tickets divided by population size), so they were excluded from the study. For the eight towns included in the study, the population sizes (P, $M = 32,424$; NP, $M = 34,839$) and median family incomes (P, $M = \$37,185$; NP, $M = \$32,220$) were not significantly different. The sales law enforcement and sales law enforcement plus fining minors intervention communities were separated geographically.

Police departments in the participating communities checked retailer compliance with local sales laws 2-3 times a year. Retailers who violated the sales laws were issued citations and fines by the court. Our research team helped communities obtain a grant from the Illinois Liquor

Control Commission (ILCC), and police departments were paid by the ILCC for conducting three rounds of compliance checks on their tobacco retailers. During the sales law enforcements, a ticket carrying a fine was issued to any merchant who sold cigarettes to a minor during a compliance check. Violations of the law were treated as a civil offense. Merchants could either pay the ticket or request an administrative hearing. Fines were about $50-$100 for the first offense, and a one-day suspension of the license to sell cigarette products plus a higher fine for a second offense. Repeated violations resulted in higher fines and longer periods of license suspensions to sell tobacco products.

For those in the P communities, minors were fined for tobacco possession. Police officers were instructed to fine minors that were caught possessing tobacco in public locations. Records of all fines were tabulated by our research staff using records from the police departments. Based on work from Woodridge, we felt that fines needed to represent above .15% of the population in the town. For example, if there were 25,000 residents, then 28 or more fines would need to be given to minors each year. The key idea is to send a message to youth that possession of tobacco is illegal, and periodic fining seems to convey this message to a community's youth. During the first year of our intervention, we were able to work with each town in the P condition to either develop or strengthen their existing ordinance so that every town in the fining minor condition had an ordinance which specified that fines could be given to minors for tobacco possession.

Rates of never use of cigarettes decreased similarly for non-white participants from 6th to 8th grades; however, for white NP participants, rates decreased 25.1%, but only 14.3% for white P participants. Occasional or everyday use increased similarly for non-whites, but for white NP youth rates increased 15.6%, but for white P youth, rates only increased 4.1%. Finally, for everyday use, a similar pattern occurred for non-white participants, but white NPs increased 6.8% and rates for white Ps increased only 2% (Jason, Pokorny, & Schoeny, 2002).

This study suggests that the combination of sales law enforcements and fines for possession decreased the percentage of smokers over time. Because a large proportion of children get tobacco from social sources, efforts focused on eliminating retail sources of tobacco may not be as effective in reducing tobacco use among youth. Possession bans may make it harder for minors to get tobacco from other minors, as fewer minors may be willing to risk the consequence of being caught with tobacco. Possession bans also make it easier to reduce subtle peer pressure when students congregate at social events and publicly smoke and encourage others to engage in this behavior.

In the present special issue, we will examine different components of this Robert Wood Johnson supported intervention. One paper will examine the types of ordinances that communities have adopted and what our recommendations are for optimal tobacco control policies at the local level. We will also examine the readiness of communities to begin the process of changing, and how that might be documented. Another domain we will investigate is whether the types of prevention programs in schools has an effect on these types of community-based interventions. We will also provide data about what influences a merchant to actually sell tobacco to minors. Finally, we will investigate whether youth who participate in these tobacco purchase efforts become more likely to try smoking or whether their attitudes change as a function of participating in these programs.

SYNTHESIS

A variety of community systems, for example, have the potential to influence the prevalence of youth smoking habits (Jason et al., 1998; Landrine, Klonoff, & Fritz, 1994). Individuals, families, schools, police, retailers, and ordinances interact in complex and dynamic ways to affect youth access to tobacco and youth smoking behaviors. At one level, for example, ordinances within the community that restrict the sale of tobacco to minors send an unambiguous message that has the potential to influence various systems within the community. Whether or not these ordinances are able to engender behavioral change (i.e., a reduction in youth access to tobacco) may very well be contingent upon the support of other systems within the community (Cummings et al., 1998). When other intervention forces act in confluence with legislation (e.g., police enforcement of tobacco-related ordinances; the provision of vendor education to increase awareness of ordinances; tobacco education in schools through special programs; the utilization of local health departments for tobacco-related projects and dissemination of health information to families and individuals, etc.), a powerful synergistic message concerning the reduction of youth access to tobacco may be activated (Jason et al., 2000).

Effective programs are more likely to be comprehensive, sustainable, well planned, and coordinated at the local level. These qualities, in turn, can significantly impact the modification of community norms and values. Prevention programs are more likely to achieve continuity when community members are involved and the program is responsive to the community's needs and resources. When efforts are sustained and long-standing, positive program impact and program outcomes can be realized.

It is increasingly being recognized that a key to comprehensive, community-oriented tobacco control policies involve enhancing local government's ability to change community norms so that youth tobacco use is seen as unacceptable. It is clear that government strategies are less costly than more individual oriented interventions, as they can reach an entire population, but it is presently unclear how to encourage communities to adopt effective anti-smoking policies. There is a need to understand successful strategies that help communities enact and enforce their local tobacco control initiatives. Change agents, such as the police officers, school officials, and other concerned anti-smoking groups, and investigators, are catalysts and facilitators of policy adoption. By gaining support from community members, our social and community interventions are more likely to be maintained over time.

At a broader level, there is a need to understand how anti-smoking norms are formed and transmitted, and to evaluate universal interventions that both reduce youth access to tobacco products and promote tobacco-free norms through taxation of tobacco products, regulation of tobacco products, enforcement of youth access laws, constraints on advertising and promotion, and tobacco control advocacy for tobacco-free environments. The authors believe that the most effective approaches will involve these types of universal interventions. The best strategies will probably involve a combination of tools including: price increases; enforcement of youth access laws; constraints on advertising and promotion; comprehensive, validated school-based programs; and media campaigns (Jason, Biglan, & Katz, 1998).

REFERENCES

Altman, D.G., Wheelis, A.Y., McFarlane, M., Lee, H., & Fortmann, S.P. (1999). The relationship between tobacco access and use among adolescents: A four community study. *Social Science and Medicine, 48,* 759-775.

Biglan, A., Henderson, J., Humphrey, D., Yasui, M., Whisman, R., Black, C., & James, L. (1995). Mobilizing positive reinforcement to reduce youth access to tobacco. *Tobacco Control, 4,* 42-48.

Centers for Disease Control. (1996). *State Tobacco Control Highlights–1996.* (CDC Publication No. 099-4895). Atlanta: National Center for Chronic Disease Prevention and Health Promotion, Office on Smoking and Health.

Chaloupka, F.J. & Pacula, R.L. (1998, Feb.). Limiting youth access to tobacco: The early impact of the Synar amendment on youth smoking. Paper presented at the 3rd Biennial Pacific Rim Allied Economic Organizations Conference, Bangkok, Thailand.

Cummings, K.M., Hyland, A., Saunders-Martin, T., Perla, J., Coppola, P.R., & T. Pechacek. (1998). Evaluation of an enforcement program to reduce tobacco sales to minors. *American Journal of Public Health, 88,* 932-936.

DiFranza, J. R., Carlson, R., & Caisse, R. (1992). Reducing youth access to tobacco. *Tobacco Control, 1,* 58.

Feighery, M. S., Altman, D. G., & Shaffer, M. A. (1991). The effects of combining education and enforcement to reduce tobacco sales to minors. *Journal of the American Medical Association, 266,* 3168-3171.

Forster, J.L., Komro, K.A., & Wolfson, M. (1996). Survey of city ordinances and local enforcement regarding commercial availability of tobacco to minors in Minnesota, United States. *Tobacco Control, 5,* 46-51.

Forster, J.L., Murray, D.M., Wolfson, M., Blaine, T.M, & Wagenaar, A.C., & Hennrikus, D.J. (1998). The effects of community policies to reduce youth access to tobacco. *American Journal of Public Health, 88,* 1193-1198.

Forster, J.L. & Wolfson, M. (1998). Youth access to tobacco: Policies and politics. *Annual Review of Public Health, 19,* 203-235.

Hinds, M. W. (1992). Impact of a local ordinance banning tobacco sales to minors. *Public Health Reports, 107,* 355-358.

Jason, L.A., Berk, M., Schnopp-Wyatt, D.L., & Talbot, B. (1999). Effects of enforcement of youth access laws on smoking prevalence. *American Journal of Community Psychology, 27,* 143-160.

Jason, L.A., Biglan, A., & Katz, R. (1998). Implications of the tobacco settlement for the prevention of teenage smoking. *Children's Services: Social Policy, Research, and Practice, 1,* 63-82.

Jason, L.A., Engstrom, M. D., Pokorny, S.B., Tegart, G., & Curie, C.J. (2000). Putting the community back into prevention: Think locally, act globally. *The Journal of Primary Prevention, 21,* 25-29.

Jason, L. A., Ji, P. Y., Anes, M., & Birkhead, S. H. (1991). Active enforcement of cigarette control laws in the prevention of cigarette sales to minors. *Journal of American Medical Association, 266* (22), 3159-3161.

Jason, L.A., Pokorny, S.B., & Schoeny, M. E. (2002). Evaluating the Effects of Enforcements and Fines on Youth Smoking. Manuscript submitted for publication.

Johnston, L.D. (1996). Cigarette smoking continues to rise among American teenagers in 1996. Ann Arbor: The University of Michigan Press.

Johnston, L. D., O'Malley, P. M., & Bachman, J. G. (1998). *Monitoring the future study, 1998.* (www.isr.umich.edu/src/mtf).

Landrine, H., Klonoff, E.A., & Fritz, J. M. (1994). Preventing cigarette sales to minors: The need for contextual sociocultural analysis. *Preventive Medicine, 23,* 322-327.

Pierce, J. P., Fiore, M. C., Novotny, T. E., Hatziandreu, E. J., & Davis, R. M. (1989). Trends in cigarette smoking in the United States, projections to the year 2000. *Journal of the American Medical Association, 261*, 65-65.

Rhodes, J. E. & Jason, L. A. (1988). *Preventing substance abuse among children & adolescents.* New York: Pergamon Press.

Rigotti, N.A., DiFranza, J.R., Chang, Y., Tisdale, T., Kemp, B., & Singer, D.E. (1997). The effect of enforcing tobacco sales laws on youths' access to tobacco and smoking behavior. *New England Journal of Medicine, 337*, 1044-1051.

Stanton, W. R., Mahalski, P. A., McGee, R., & Silva, P. A. (1993). Reasons for smoking or not smoking in adolescence. *Addictive Behavior, 18*, 321-329.

Strouse, R. & Hall, J. (1994). *Robert Wood Johnson Foundation youth access survey: Results of a national household survey to assess public attitudes about policy alternatives for limiting minor's access to tobacco products* (26023): Mathematical Policy Research, Inc.

Talbot, B. (1992). "Adolescent smokers' rights laws." *Tobacco Control, 1*, 294-295.

Unger, J.B., Rohrbach, L.A., Howard, K.A., Cruz, T.B., Johnson, C.A., & Chen, X. (1999). Attitudes toward anti-tobacco policy among California youth: Associations with smoking status, psychosocial variables and advocacy actions. *Health Education Research, 14*, 751-763.

Measuring the Quality of Laws Limiting Youth Access to Tobacco

Steven B. Pokorny
Leonard A. Jason
Heidi Lautenschlager
Rhonda Smith

DePaul University

Stephanie M. Townsend

University of Illinois at Chicago

SUMMARY. In response to the prevalence of tobacco use by minors, policy makers have sought more effective ways to use public policy to reduce tobacco use initiation and consumption and to promote smoking cessation. While various tools are available for assessing tobacco control laws, they are limited by a narrow focus on retail sales and omit many components of a comprehensive, ecological approach to tobacco control. This article presents a measure for rating laws designed to control youth access to tobacco. The measure evaluates components of laws pertaining to retailer licensing, tobacco sales to minors and compliance with sales

---

Address correspondence to: Steven B. Pokorny, PhD, Youth Tobacco Access Project, Center for Community Research, DePaul University, 990 W. Fullerton Avenue, Chicago, IL 60614.

The authors express appreciation for financial support provided by The Robert Wood Johnson Foundation.

[Haworth co-indexing entry note]: "Measuring the Quality of Laws Limiting Youth Access to Tobacco." Pokorny, Steven B. et al. Co-published simultaneously in *Journal of Prevention & Intervention in the Community* (The Haworth Press, Inc.) Vol. 24, No. 1, 2002, pp. 15-27; and: *Preventing Youth Access to Tobacco* (ed: Leonard A. Jason, and Steven B. Pokorny) The Haworth Press, Inc., 2002, pp. 15-27. Single or multiple copies of this article are available for a fee from The Haworth Document Delivery Service [1-800-HAWORTH 9:00 a.m. - 5:00 p.m. (EST). E-mail address: getinfo@haworthpressinc.com].

15

laws, distribution and location of tobacco products, and youth possession of tobacco. Data are presented that indicate the measure can detect
differences in the comprehensiveness of tobacco control laws and that it
is a reliable measure. *[Article copies available for a fee from The Haworth
Document Delivery Service: 1-800-HAWORTH. E-mail address: <getinfo@
haworthpressinc.com> Website: <http://www.HaworthPress.com> © 2002 by
The Haworth Press, Inc. All rights reserved.]*

KEYWORDS. Minors, tobacco, laws, youth access, illegal sales

Tobacco use by minors is a pervasive societal problem in the United
States with significant health and economic consequences to both the
individuals affected and the public. Recent population estimates indicate that each day in the United States 4,800 youth try smoking for the
first time and almost 3,000 more become established smokers (Gilpin,
Choice, Berry, & Pierce, 1999). In response to the prevalence of tobacco use by minors, policy makers have sought more effective ways to
use public policy in reducing tobacco use initiation and consumption
and to promote smoking cessation. The power of policy stems from its
environmental approach that allows for relatively small changes in legislation and enforcement behavior to have a large public health impact
(Jason, Biglan, & Katz, 1998). Therefore, policy initiatives for tobacco
control are proposed to be immediate, inexpensive and powerful ways
to impact adolescent tobacco use. One of the controversial issues in the
regulation of tobacco use is the balance between individuals' freedom
to use tobacco legally with society's obligation to limit the usage of le-
thal products (Jacobson, Wassermen, & Anderson, 1997). Fortunately,
there is strong public support among both smokers and nonsmokers for
the implementation and enforcement of laws that restrict youth access
to tobacco (Jeffrey et al., 1990).

There is evidence that tobacco control legislation is an effective way
to impact the smoking behavior of youth. A longitudinal, statewide
study conducted in Massachusetts found that youth living in towns with
local tobacco legislation were less likely to become established smokers
than youth living in towns without a local ordinance (Siegel, Biener, &
Rigotti, 1999). Additionally, a study in Minnesota assisted communities in an intervention group in developing local tobacco control ordinances and found that while both the intervention and control communities showed an increase in youth smoking, communities with local or-

dinances showed a significantly lower net prevalence of youth smoking (Forster et al., 1998). Four broad policy areas that may be important for tobacco control are the licensing of tobacco retailers, tobacco sales to minors and compliance with sales laws, the distribution and location of tobacco products, and youth possession of tobacco. Each of these areas is discussed below.

Retailer licenses are a process by which a municipality requires the annual renewal of a paid license for all retailers who sell tobacco products, whether over-the-counter or through a vending machine. Suspension or revocation of a license, even temporarily, can result in a greater impact on retailer revenues than even a moderate fine, thereby creating a more substantial incentive for retailers to implement policies and procedures to minimize illegal tobacco sales in their places of business. Additionally, the cost of annual renewal of licenses can help to fund the municipality's tobacco sales enforcement operations. Therefore, even if no retailer is fined for illegally selling tobacco to a minor, the municipality is still ensured an annual source of revenue for funding compliance checks. Additionally, by limiting the number of licenses available, the municipality can reduce the availability and visibility of tobacco in the community. Retailer licensing has been shown to be an important component in reducing cigarette sales rates to minors to a minimal level and in reducing cigarette experimentation and regular smoking among youth (Jason, Ji, Anes, & Birkhead, 1991; Jason, Berk, Schnopp-Wyatt, & Talbot, 1999).

A comprehensive approach to limiting tobacco sales to minors extends beyond prohibiting the sale of tobacco products to persons under the age of 18 years and includes six aspects of sales to minors. First, the prohibition of the sale of tobacco products to persons under the age of 18 years can deter current smoking and intent to smoke among minors (Lewit, Hyland, Kerrebrock, & Cummings, 1997) Second, setting the minimum legal age to purchase tobacco at 18 years allows for the prosecution of minors who attempt to purchase tobacco. Third, in light of evidence that retailers who request age or photo identification make fewer illegal tobacco sales to minors (Arday et al., 1997; Curie, Pokorny, Jason, Schoeny, & Townsend, 2002; DiFranza, Savageua, & Aisquit, 1996), requiring merchants to request photo identification for customers who appear younger than 21 years of age can decrease the likelihood of illegal sales based on mistaken age assessments. Fourth, the prohibition against persons under the age of 18 years from misrepresenting their age or using any false or altered identification for the purpose of purchasing tobacco products can decrease the likelihood of retailers being deceived about a customer's age. Fifth, requiring the posting of warning signs regarding sales to minors at the point of sale of tobacco products serves as a public reminder to both retailers and customers of the sales laws. Finally, allowing for the publication of the names of outlets that make illegal sales to minors can increase parental awareness of where youth may go to purchase tobacco and stimulate public pressure on retailers that illegally sell tobacco and public reinforcement for those retailers who do not.

In addition to prohibitions and requirements related to tobacco sales to minors, enforcement of the sales laws is necessary for reducing the sales rate to minors (Gemson et al., 1998; Rigotti et al., 1997). There are five issues related to enforcement of the minimum age of sales laws. First, the designation of a local agency that is primarily responsible for the enforcement of the law banning sales to minors can eliminate bureaucratic complications regarding enforcement responsibilities. Second, the requirement of annual, random, unannounced inspections of over-the-counter and vending machine tobacco sales can ensure that retailers will undergo a minimum number of inspections. Typically, these inspections are conducted with the assistance of underage youth who are paid to attempt to purchase tobacco under the supervision of the enforcement agency. Third, allowing for the owners or licensees to be held accountable for the actions of their employees can provide additional incentive for people in management positions to train their employees in how to avoid illegal sales and to implement procedures that reduce the likelihood of illegal sales. Fourth, the establishment of civil penalties (e.g., fines, license suspensions, etc.) rather than criminal penalties for those who violate the sales laws can increase the rate of enforcement since civil penalties generally require fewer prosecutorial resources and are usually met with less opposition from the community. The final provision involves the use of a graduated system of fines and license suspensions or revocations for retailers that sell tobacco products to minors and allows for greater accountability for repeat offenders.

In considering the mode of distribution and the location of tobacco products in stores, there are six issues pertaining to youth access to tobacco. First, the prohibition against persons under the age of 18 years from selling tobacco products is an attempt to reduce the pressure on teenage employees to sell tobacco to their peers who may exploit the peer relationship in attempting to purchase tobacco. Second, the ban on the sale of tobacco products within a specified distance from schools, child care facilities, or other educational/recreational facilities used by minors is aimed at reducing the amount youth are exposed to tobacco advertising and to make retail tobacco less accessible to youth. Third, limitations on tobacco/cigarette vending machines are a response to the easy access presented by vending machines. The most effective deterrent to youth access is a ban on all vending machines, regardless of location or locking device; however, the presence of a lock on vending machines presents at least a nominal deterrent (DiFranza et al., 1996; Forster et al., 1992). Fourth, the prohibition on the sale of tobacco products by self-service displays and the requirement that all tobacco products be kept in a locked case are associated with lower illegal sales rates to minors (Widley, Woodruff, Pamplone, & Conway, 1995) and can reduce the physical access to tobacco that facilitates shoplifting. DiFranza, Eddy, Brown, Ryan, and Bogojavlensky (1994) found that as many as 50 percent of young smokers admit to shoplifting tobacco at least once, and they suggest that shoplifting may become more prevalent as it becomes more difficult for youth to purchase tobacco. Fifth, the prohibition of the sale of cigarettes individually or in packages of less than 20 cigarettes and the ban on the distribution of free tobacco samples, coupons for free tobacco samples, or rebates (Lewit et al., 1997) can reduce the economic accommodation of youths' limited financial resources that these small size sales represent. The final provision provides for the ban on tobacco look-alike products (e.g., candy cigarettes, chewing gum packaged like chewing tobacco, etc.) and is an effort to reduce early reinforcement of tobacco use behavior among youth, including young children.

Penalizing youth for possessing tobacco is a controversial issue in which the tobacco industry is usually found in favor of such penalties and anti-tobacco advocates are usually found opposed to such penalties because of a perception that they relieve the industry of responsibility for youth smoking. Based on previous research (Jason et al., 1991; Jason et al., 1999), it is hypothesized that communities that actively enforce youth possession laws will show a greater reduction in youth tobacco use than communities that only enforce minimum age of sales laws due to a deterrent effect of the possession laws on experimental tobacco use.

While various tools are available for assessing tobacco control laws (Alciati et al., 1998; Klonoff et al., 1998), they are limited by a narrow focus on retail sales and the omission of many of the issues identified above. The measure developed by Alciati et al. (1998) assesses how extensive state laws are in reducing youth access to tobacco by rating tobacco control laws on nine items: minimum age of sales, packaging, clerk intervention, photo identification, vending machines, free distributions, graduated penalties, random inspections, and statewide enforcement. With the exception of statewide enforcement, these items can also be used to assess municipal ordinances. For each item, a target was specified that reflected public health objectives and ratings were completed based on the extent to which the target was met or exceeded. Ratings ranged from five ("exceeds target") to zero ("no effective provision").

While the simplicity of the measure facilitates ease of implementation, the lack of more specificity in the measure is a challenge when assessing a large number of statutes that lack uniformity. Additionally, the measure omits any assessment of the following tobacco control provisions: retailer licensing system, limitations on the number of tobacco outlets, establishing the minimum age to purchase tobacco at 18 years or older, prohibitions against minors misrepresenting their age or using false or altered identification for the purpose of purchasing tobacco, the publication of the names of retailers that make illegal sales to minors, allowing for the owner or licensee to be held accountable for the actions of employees, prohibitions against minors selling tobacco products, requirements that tobacco products be kept in a locked case, prohibitions against tobacco look-alike products, and any provisions concerning youth possession of tobacco.

The Assessment of the Comprehensiveness of Tobacco Laws Scale (Act-L Scale) developed by Klonoff et al. (1998) assesses tobacco control laws on 55 items. The Act-L Scale is divided into three subscales: environmental tobacco smoke, tobacco advertising and promotion, and youth access to tobacco. Each item is treated as a dichotomous variable with raters indicating that a law either does or does not contain specific provisions for tobacco control. The number of items included in the statute are summed to yield a score out of a possible total of 55 points. Statutes with a higher score are considered to be more comprehensive than statutes with a lower score. This measure is particularly useful to municipalities since it was developed to be used by individuals who have no prior training in the law or in tobacco control issues. With appropriate training on how to use the scale, raters should be able to rate statutes with a high degree of reliability.

While youth access subscale of the ACT-L Scale is more comprehensive than Alciati et al.'s measure, it also omits numerous provisions, including: requiring retailers to request photographic identification for customers who appear younger than the age of 21 years, prohibiting minors from misrepresenting their age or using any false or altered identification for the purpose of purchasing tobacco, allowing for the owner or licensee to be held accountable for the actions of employees, prohibiting minors from selling tobacco, and any provisions concerning youth possession of tobacco.

In an effort to assist communities in controlling youth access to tobacco, a research group at DePaul University developed a measure for assessing the comprehensiveness of both state and municipal tobacco control laws. For over 12 years, the research group has been investigating methods of reducing youth access to tobacco at a community level (Jason et al., 1991; Jason et al., 1999). The current project is the Youth Tobacco Access Project (YTAP), which is a three-year, randomized trial, multi-community intervention designed to examine the effectiveness of both sales and possession enforcement strategies in reducing youth access to tobacco. Across both experimental and control communities, the project assumes an active intervention component. In response to community requests for assistance in strengthening their local tobacco control ordinances, the research team developed a measure for assessing the comprehensiveness of tobacco control laws that identifies the components of tobacco control policy that need to be added to an existing law in order to have a larger impact on youth behavior. The present study presents the measure for evaluating laws designed to control youth access to tobacco and analyzes inter-rater reliability for the measure.

METHODS

Participants

Sixty-three towns in northern and central Illinois participated in the present study. Town populations ranged from 122 to 99,581 ($M = 16,218$, $SD = 20,264$), with the percentage of the population under age 18 years ranging from .04 to .35 ($M = .25$, $SD = .05$) (U.S. Census Bureau, 1990). The median income for participating towns ranged from $20,328 to $83,353 ($M = $37,218$, $SD = $11,949$), and the percentage of the population with more than a high school education ranged from .55 to .95 ($M = .77$, $SD = .11$) (U.S. Census Bureau, 1990).

Materials

The scale used in this study to assess the comprehensiveness of tobacco control laws was generated from two other rating scales: the Assessment of the Comprehensiveness of Tobacco Laws Scale (Act-L Scale) (Klonoff et al., 1998) and a rating system developed by Alciati et al. (1998). In addition to items taken from these scales, additional items were added to include policy initiatives that were not present in the ACT-L Scale and Alciati et al.'s scale. The resulting measure, the Assessment of the Comprehensiveness of Youth Tobacco Control Laws, assesses tobacco retailer licensing (3 items), tobacco sales to minors and compliance with sales laws (13 items), distribution and location of tobacco products (8 items), and youth possession of tobacco (3 items) (See Appendix A). Items are rated dichotomously as either "yes" or "no," with a "yes" indicating that the law being assessed includes that item. Each "yes" rating is equivalent to one point, with the sum score yielding a possible total of 28 points.

Procedure

City officials in 68 urban, suburban, and rural municipalities in northern and central Illinois received a letter requesting copies of all tobacco-related ordinances for their jurisdiction. Municipalities were selected based on their involvement in the larger study of the Youth Tobacco Access Project (11 towns) or their proximity to those 11 towns. Of the local ordinances received, 45% were initially returned while 55% required further contact. Follow-up phone calls were done until 63 out of the 68 town officials complied with the request. This reflects a total return rate of 93%. The towns that did not respond were rural communities within 30 miles of each other. Of the 63 towns that responded, officials in 38 towns returned a local tobacco-control policy while officials in 25 towns reported following the Illinois State statutes concerning tobacco control.

Two undergraduate volunteers who had no formal legal education were trained during a two-hour session in which they independently evaluated mock ordinances using the Assessment of the Comprehensiveness of Youth Tobacco Control Laws. The purpose of using mock ordinances was to familiarize raters with typical legal language and policy formats. The rating of mock ordinances continued until the raters reached 100% agreement on their ratings, resulting in the rating of three mock ordinances. Following the training, the raters proceeded independently to rate the tobacco control ordinances for the 38 towns with local ordinances plus the Illinois State statutes pertaining to tobacco control.

RESULTS

Ratings for the 38 local ordinances and the Illinois State statutes pertaining to tobacco control ranged from scores of 2 points to 17 points out of a possible total of 28 points ($M = 9.25$, $SD = 3.9$). The ratings were analyzed using Cohen's Kappa to determine inter-rater reliability, resulting in a range from 0.64 to 1.00 ($M = 0.90$, $SD = 0.09$). These findings indicate that the Assessment of the Comprehensiveness of Youth Tobacco Control Laws can detect differences in the comprehensiveness of different municipal and state laws and that it is a reliable measure.

DISCUSSION

In this article, a measure for assessing laws to control youth access to tobacco was described that assessed retailer licensing, tobacco sales to minors and compliance with sales laws, distribution and location of tobacco products, and youth possession of tobacco. The measure was developed as a resource for communities that are seeking to adopt a municipal tobacco control ordinance or to strengthen an existing ordinance. The strength of this measure is its comprehensive, ecological approach to youth access to tobacco. To a greater degree than other measures, the scale described here assesses multiple strategies to change community norms. Consequently, it can be used by communities and states to assess existing laws and to direct future legislative action. Its limitation is that empirical support does not yet exist for all components of the scale. Further study employing controlled experimental design is needed to substantiate the items in the present scale.

The most substantial threat to municipal tobacco control ordinances is state preemption, which is advocated by the tobacco industry and opposed by many public health professionals and associations (Alciati et al., 1998). A 1998 survey of all 50 states found that 15 states preempt licensing ordinances, 12 states preempt minor sales ordinances, 8 states preempt youth possession ordinances, and 11 states preempt advertising ordinances (Gardiner et al., 2000). State preemption of municipal ordinances weakens and limits policy approaches to the problem of youth access to tobacco by eliminating municipalities as a testing ground for policies, eliminating information regarding the costs and benefits of different policy approaches, and curtailing local debate over ordinances that can stimulate education on youth tobacco use in the community (Alciati et al., 1998). Preemption also complicates policy analyses due to "grandfather" clauses and universal versus specific pre-emption (Gardiner et al., 2000). Additionally, preemption removes incentives for local enforcement initiatives. Many states require that fines issued under state laws be divided between the state and the local prosecuting agency. In contrast, fines issued under municipal ordinances remain in the local community and can be used to fund further enforcement operations. As more states move to preempt municipal control ordinances, it is to the benefit of local communities to adopt ordinances in an expedient manner. By adopting ordinances with haste, municipalities may be able to avert preemptive action by being "grandfathered" in, thereby bypassing state preemptive actions.

It is important to recognize that the adoption and enforcement of a municipal ordinance is not sufficient to eliminate youth access to tobacco or to exert a significant impact on the prevalence of youth tobacco use. Communities need to employ multiple strategies for reducing youth tobacco use that include the enforcement of policies to reduce youth access to tobacco, media advocacy, youth anti-tobacco activities, family communications, and school-based interventions (Biglan et al., 1996). Municipal and state laws that restrict youth access to tobacco and youth possession of tobacco are a vital component of a community-wide approach, as they send an unambiguous message that tobacco use by youth is not tolerated. When supported by other community systems, tobacco control policies have the potential to stimulate behavioral change and reduce the prevalence of youth tobacco use.

REFERENCES

Alciati, M. H., Frosh, M., Green, S. B., Brownson, R. C., Fisher, P. H., Hobart, R., Roman, A., Sciandra, R. C., & Shelton, D. M. (1998). State laws on youth access to tobacco in the United States: Measuring their extensiveness with a new rating system. *Tobacco Control, 7,* 345-352.

Arday, D. R., Klevens, R. M., Nelson, D. E., Huang, P., Giovino, G. A., & Mowrey, P. (1997). Predictors of tobacco sales to minors. *Preventive Medicine, 26,* 8-13.

Biglan, A., Ary, D. V., Yudelson, H., Duncan, T. E., Hood, D. James, L., Koehn, V., Wright, Z., Black, C., Levings, D., Smith, S., & Graiser, E. (1996). Experimental evaluation of a modular approach to mobilizing antitobacco influences of peers and parents. *American Journal of Community Psychology, 24,* 311-339.

Curie, C. J., Pokorny, S. B., Jason, L. A., Schoeny, M., & Townsend, S. M. (2002). An examination of factors influencing illegal tobacco sales to minors. *Journal of Prevention & Intervention in the Community, 24,* 63-76.

DiFranza, J. R., Eddy, J. J., Brown, L. F., Ryan, J. L., & Bogajavlensky, A. (1994). Tobacco acquisition and cigarette brand selection among youth. *Tobacco Control, 4,* 334-338.

DiFranza, J. R., Savageau, J. A., & Aisquith, B. F. (1996). Youth access to tobacco: The effects of age, gender, vending machine locks, and "It's the Law" programs. *American Journal of Public Health, 864,* 221-224.

Forster, J. L., Murray, D. M., Wolfson, M., Blaine, T. M., Wagenaar, A. C., & Hennrikus, D. J. (1998). The effects of community policies to reduce youth access to tobacco. *American Journal of Public Health, 88,* 1193-1198.

Gardiner, J. A., Kuhns, L. M., Hubrich, J., & Kreps, B. (2000). Local governments and tobacco control policies: Role variations and sources of data [On-line]. Available: www.uic.edu/departs/ossr/impacteen.

Gemson, D. H., Moats, H. L., Watkins, B. X., Ganze, M. L., Robinson, S., & Healton, E. (1998). Laying down the law: Reducing illegal tobacco sales to minors in central Harlem. *American Journal of Public Health, 88,* 936-939.

Gilpin, E. A., Choi, W. S., Berry, C., & Pierce, J. P. (1999). How many adolescents start smoking each day in the United States? *Journal of Adolescent Health, 25,* 248-255.

Jacobson, P. D., Wassermen, J., & Anderson, J.R. (1997). The politics of antismoking legislation: Lessons from six states. *Journal of Health Politics, Policy and Law, 18,* 787-819.

Jason, L.A., Berk, M., Schnopp-Wyatt, D.L., & Talbot, B. (1999). Effects of enforcement of youth access laws on smoking prevalence. *American Journal of Community Psychology, 27,* 143-160.

Jason, L. A., Biglan, A., & Katz, R. (1998). Implications of the tobacco settlement for the prevention of teenage smoking. *Children's Services: Social Policy, Research, and Practice, 1,* 63-82.

Jason, L. A., Ji, P. Y., Anes, M., & Birkhead, S. H. (1991). Active enforcement of cigarette control laws in the prevention of cigarette sales to minors. *Journal of American Medical Association, 266,* 3159-3161.

Jeffrey, R. W., Forster, J. L., Schmid, T. L., McBride, C. M., Rooney, B. L., & Pirie, P. L. (1990). Community attitudes toward public policies to control alcohol, tobacco, and high-fat food consumption. *American Journal of Preventive Medicine, 6,* 12-19.

Klonoff, E. A., Landrine, H., Alcaraz, R., Campbell, R. R., Lang, D. L., McSwan, K. L., Parekh, B., & Norton-Perry, G. (1998). An instrument for assessing the quality of tobacco-control policies: The ACT-L Scale. *Preventive Medicine, 27,* 808-814.

Lewit, E. M., Hyland, A., Kerrebrock, N., & Cummings, K. M. (1997). Price, public policy, and smoking in young people. *Tobacco Control, 6,* S17-S24.

National Cancer Institute. (1993). Model Sale of Tobacco to Minors Ordinance. *Smoking and tobacco control, 3: Major local tobacco control ordinances in the United States.* (NIH No. 93-3532).

Rigotti, N. A., DiFranza, J. R., Chang, Y., Tisdale, T., Kemp, B., & Singer, D. E. (1997). The effect of enforcing tobacco-sales laws on adolescents' access to tobacco and smoking behavior. *New England Journal of Medicine, 37,* 1044-1051.

Siegel, M., Biener, L., & Rigotti, N. A. (1999). The effect of local tobacco sales laws on adolescent smoking initiation. *Preventive Medicine, 29*, 334-342.

U. S. Census Bureau. (1990). *United States Census, 1990* [On-line]. Available: factfinder.census.gov.

U. S. Department of Health and Human Services. (1994). *Preventing tobacco use among young people: A report of the Surgeon General.* Atlanta: U. S. Department of Health and Human Services.

Widley, M. B., Woodruff, S. I., Pamplone, S. Z., & Conway, T. L. (1995). Self-service sale of tobacco: How it contributes to youth access. *Tobacco Control, 4*, 355-361.

APPENDIX A
Assessment of the Comprehensiveness of Youth Tobacco Control Laws

Assessment of the Comprehensiveness of Youth Tobacco Control Laws

DATE_____   EVALUATOR CODE_____
CITY CODE_____   DATE (S) OF THE LAW(S)_____ _____ _____

Instructions: Put a check mark (next to "yes" or "no") in the space that best describes the law.

DOES THE LAW...

Licensing

1) Include a merchant licensing system to sell tobacco	YES___	NO___
2) Limit the number of licensed tobacco outlets	YES___	NO___
3) Provide for the suspension or revocation of the license for violations of the tobacco law/ordinance	YES___	NO___

Sales to minors/compliance

4) Prohibit the **sale** of tobacco products to persons under the age of eighteen	YES___	NO___
5) Set the minimum legal age to **purchase** tobacco at 18 years or older	YES___	NO___
6) Require merchants to request photographic identification for customers who appear younger than the age of 21	YES___	NO___
7) Prohibit persons under the age of eighteen from misrepresenting their age or using any false or altered identification for the purpose of purchasing tobacco products	YES___	NO___
8) Require the posting of warning signs regarding **sales to minors** at the point of sale of tobacco products	YES___	NO___
9) Include the publication of the names of outlets that make illegal sales to minors	YES___	NO___
10) Designate a local agency that will be primarily responsible for enforcement of the law banning sales to minors	YES___	NO___
11) Include annual, random, unannounced inspections of over-the-counter tobacco sales	YES___	NO___
12) Include annual, random, unannounced inspections of vending machine tobacco sales	YES___	NO___
13) Allow for the owner or licensee to be held accountable for the actions of his employees	YES___	NO___
14) Establish penalties applicable to persons who sell tobacco products to minors	YES___	NO___
15) Rely on civil (*e.g.,* fines, injunctions, infractions, violations of Health and Safety codes) rather than criminal penalties for those who violate the law banning sales to children	YES___	NO___
16) Include a graduated system of fines, penalties, and suspensions for merchants that sell tobacco products to minors		

APPENDIX A (continued)

(*e.g.,* 1st offense: fined $200 and notification of future fines
2nd: fined $500 and suspension of license between 90 business days and
6 mos.; 3rd: fined $1000 and revocation of license between 9 mos.
and 19 mos.)   YES___   NO___

Distribution /location of products

17) Prohibit persons under the age of 18 from **selling** tobacco products   YES___   NO___
18) Ban the sale of tobacco products within a specified distance from schools,
  child care facilities or other educational/recreational facilities used by minors YES___   NO___
19) Ban tobacco/cigarette vending machines except in "adult only" locations
  (e.g., bars) **or** require that vending machines be fitted with a locking device   YES___   NO___
20) Ban all tobacco/cigarette vending machines (regardless of location)   YES___   NO___
21) Prohibit the sale of tobacco products by self-service displays   YES___   NO___
22) Require that all tobacco products to be kept in a locked case   YES___   NO___
23) Prohibit the sale of cigarettes individually or in packages of less
  than 20 cigarettes   YES___   NO___
24) Ban the distribution of free tobacco samples or coupons for free tobacco
  samples or rebates   YES___   NO___
25) Ban tobacco look-alike products   YES___   NO___

Possession

26) Prohibit persons under the age of 18 from possessing tobacco products   YES___   NO___
27) Establish fines applicable to persons under the age of 18 for the possession
  of tobacco products   YES___   NO___
28) Include a graduated system of fines and penalties for persons under the
  age of 18 for possession of tobacco products
  (*e.g.,* 1st offense: fine $50 or smoking cessation program;
  2nd: fine $50-$100 and smoking cessation program;
  3rd: fine $75-$300 and smoking cessation program and community service)   YES___   NO___

Indicate any questions or problems you had evaluating this city's law:

_____
_____
_____
_____

Community Readiness for Prevention: Applying Stage Theory to Multi-Community Interventions

Mark Engstrom

University of Illinois at Chicago

Leonard A. Jason

DePaul University

Stephanie M. Townsend

University of Illinois at Chicago

Steven B. Pokorny

DePaul University

Carrie J. Curie

University of Kansas

SUMMARY. This study presents an effort to adapt the community readiness model to a multi-community intervention to reduce youth ac-

Address correspondence to: Mark Engstrom, Psychology Department, The University of Illinois at Chicago, 1007 West Harrison, Chicago, IL 60607-7137.

The authors express appreciation for financial support provided by the Robert Wood Johnson Foundation and David Altman, the National Program Director, and Andrea Williams, the Deputy Director, of the Substance Abuse Policy Research Program.

[Haworth co-indexing entry note]: "Community Readiness for Prevention: Applying Stage Theory to Multi-Community Interventions." Engstrom, Mark et al. Co-published simultaneously in *Journal of Prevention & Intervention in the Community* (The Haworth Press, Inc.) Vol. 24, No. 1, 2002, pp. 29-46; and: *Preventing Youth Access to Tobacco* (ed: Leonard A. Jason, and Steven B. Pokorny) The Haworth Press, Inc., 2002, pp. 29-46. Single or multiple copies of this article are available for a fee from The Haworth Document Delivery Service [1-800-HAWORTH 9:00 a.m. - 5:00 p.m. (EST). E-mail address: getinfo@haworthpressinc.com].

cess to tobacco. The background of the original community readiness model is outlined, and a behaviorally based adaptation specific to tobacco sales and tobacco possession enforcement is presented. Data on behaviorally based readiness ratings for 11 communities are presented. Correlational analyses indicate a significant relationship between ratings for sales enforcement readiness and the number of tobacco compliance checks conducted by the local police departments. The relationship between possession enforcement readiness and the rate of citations issued was in the expected direction, but was not significant. The results indicate that the behavioral adaptation of the community readiness model can: (a) provide a conceptual heuristic to understand community dynamics; (b) increase responsiveness to each community's unique needs; (c) measure changes over time; and (d) inform future intervention strategies with the community. *[Article copies available for a fee from The Haworth Document Delivery Service: 1-800-HAWORTH. E-mail address: <getinfo@haworthpressinc.com> Website: <http://www.HaworthPress.com> © 2002 by The Haworth Press, Inc. All rights reserved.]*

KEYWORDS. Readiness, community, tobacco, illegal sales, fining minors

Increasingly, community-based prevention efforts are being called upon to deal with a number of issues related to mental, physical, and social well-being (Donnermeyer, Plested, Edwards, Oetting, & Littlethunder, 1997; Howard-Pitney, 1990). These issues include problems related to substance abuse, sexually transmitted diseases, domestic violence and child abuse, criminal activity, homelessness, and depression, among others. The increasing popularity of locally oriented prevention strategies is a result of the demonstrated effectiveness of community approaches in areas such as health promotion, crime and delinquency prevention, and community development (Kumpfer, Whiteside, Wanderman, & Cardenas, 1997). With the proliferation of community-based efforts comes a shift in emphasis from individual factors toward the overall health and social ecology of the community (Goodman, Wanderman, Chinman, Imm, & Morrissey, 1996; Howard-Pitney, 1990). No longer solely focusing on individual-level behavior change, community-based prevention efforts have begun to consider the social and cultural contexts in which individual behaviors occur. Toward this end, there is a growing consensus that effective prevention efforts have similar underlying themes: They use a systematic approach, employ multiple methods, encourage collaboration among community groups, and consider community-level processes that contribute to normative change (Edwards, Jumper-Thurman, Plested, Oetting, & Swanson, 1999; Goodman et al., 1996; Levine, 1998). Together, these themes hold promise in revealing community dynamics critical to the success of burgeoning local preventive interventions.

As community-based prevention efforts continue to gain exposure, however, an increased awareness of the challenges associated with local approaches must be brought to bear. While the benefits of implementing successful community-based prevention programs are compelling, it is by no means a given that simply establishing such a program within a community foretells success. Many programs fail as a result of poor planning, lack of potency in changing community norms, or insufficient preparation of program staff (Edwards et al., 1999). Even after a local prevention program has been implemented, many other factors threaten its effectiveness and longevity. Some programs, for example, are not based on sound information or tested scientific theories (Donnermeyer et al., 1997), while others run out of funding before they are able to achieve desired ends.

Some of the challenges to implementing community-based programs are related to the unique characteristics of the communities themselves. Each community is comprised of its own attitudes, values, resources, history, political climate, strengths, and weaknesses (Edwards et al., 1999). These contexts can affect the trajectory of a local prevention effort, particularly when they are not considered during the planning and implementation of a program. When the characteristics of the community do not support the goals of the program, prevention programs may have to overcome additional hurdles in achieving their goals. For example, a community program whose goal is to reduce unwanted pregnancies by introducing a controversial method of birth control may be met by resistance if the attitudes and values of the community are inconsistent with the program's approach. Such a program may be doomed to failure, or, at least, a reduced set of desirable outcomes. Prevention programs can improve their chances for success through appropriate planning that takes into account the unique characteristics that distinguish communities from one another; they can then adapt program goals and methods based upon the nature of those characteristics.

Given the impact that community-level factors often have upon the effectiveness of locally based interventions, and because of the increased implementation of these interventions, there has been a need to articulate systematically the challenges that are present when establishing a program that intends to deal with a community-specific problem (Edwards et al., 1999). There has also been a need to develop methods to overcome these challenges and make progress toward the goals of the program. Community readiness theory, developed by Oetting et al. (1995), was developed to meet these needs (Donnermeyer et al., 1997; Edwards et al., 1999; Edwards, Jumper-Thurman, Plested, Oetting, & Swanson, 2000; Jumper-Thurman, Plested, Edwards, & Oetting, 1998; Plested, Smithman, Jumper-Thurman, Oetting, & Edwards, 1999; Plested, Jumper-Thurman, Edwards, & Oetting, 1998). These researchers note that the community readiness model can be used to assess a community's readiness for prevention programming. This assessment, in turn, provides a basis for understanding the relationship between community dynamics and the program and suggests methods to overcome prevention hurdles based upon the assessment (Plested et al., 1999).

Although the original community readiness model was developed for use with alcohol and drug abuse prevention programs, the broader aim in its creation was in suggesting methods in which the assessment of community readiness can be applied to a variety of community-based prevention efforts (Oetting et al., 1995).

THEORETICAL BACKGROUND

More and more, community researchers are discovering that communities vary widely in their interest, willingness, and competence in engaging in prevention efforts (Goodman et al., 1996; Oetting et al., 1995). Some communities deny that a problem exists in their community. Other communities may have recognized that a community problem exists and have already developed methods to deal with it. Most communities probably fall somewhere in between these extremes (Kumpfer et al., 1997). They may be aware of a problem within the community but possess little knowledge of what to do about it, or they may have a program that is up and running that has been unable to attain its goals. A significant challenge in initiating a community-based prevention program is to determine a community's level of readiness to engage in activity related to the goals of the prevention program.

The idea of assessing community readiness shares features with concepts that focus attention on the environments in which prevention activity occurs. These include the ecological principle of adaptation, which describes how environments shape the behaviors that occur within them (Burgoyne & Jason, 1991; Goodman et al., 1996; Kelly, 1968). Other concepts describe the significance of community motivation (Hallman & Wandersman, 1992); community identity (Puddifoot, 1995; Puddifoot, 1996); community or organizational climate (Butterfoss, Goodman, & Wandersman, 1996); community interest (Schooler & Flora, 1997); systems thinking (Fuqua, Newman, & Dickman, 1999); and the perception of positive and negative aspects of the community environment (Chavis & Wandersman, 1990).

Community readiness theory is "based on the underlying premises that: (1) communities are at different stages of readiness for dealing with a specific problem, (2) that the stage of readiness can be accurately assessed, (3) that communities can be moved through a series of stages to develop, implement, maintain, and improve effective programs, and (4) that it is critical to identify the stage of readiness because interventions to move communities to the next stage differ for each stage of readiness" (Edwards et al., 1999, paragraph 11). The development of these stages and the model itself has been informed by two separate yet related processes: psychological readiness for treatment and community development (Donnermeyer et al., 1997; Jumper Thurman et al., 1999; Oetting et al., 1995). Created for use in describing people with addictive behaviors, the model of psychological readiness for treatment demonstrated that individual readiness was a critical factor in the successful initiation and implementation of psychotherapeutic treatment (Edwards et al., 1999; Prochaska, DiClemente, & Norcross, 1992). Prochaska, DiClemente and Norcross (1992) describe five stages of change in individuals: (a) *precontemplation*–no intention to change behavior and a lack of awareness of problem; (b) *contemplation*–awareness of problem but no commitment to take action; (c) *preparation*–intention to take action; (d) *action*–implementation of desired behavior change; and (e) *maintenance*–consolidation of gains achieved through the action stage and prevention of relapse to earlier stages (Prochaska et al., 1992). While this model provided a useful analogue, it did not provide a sufficient number of stages to reflect the multidimensional and group processes necessary for a comprehensive model of community readiness.

From the field of community development, community readiness theory draws from two parallel processes: Beal's (1964) *social action process* and Rogers' (1983) *diffusion of innovations* model. Beal's social action process describes the initiation and legitimization of change within a community by using five stages (Donnermeyer et al., 1997;

Oetting et al., 1995): (a) *stimulation of interest*–the recognition of need for a new idea within the community; (b) *initiation*–the proposal and promotion of a new idea by community members; (c) *legitimization*–the decision by community members to do something; (d) *decision to act*–the development of a specific plan of action; and (e) *action*–the implementation of a plan of action. Rogers' (1983) diffusion of innovations model describes the *innovation decision-making process*, which also includes five stages: (a) *knowledge*–an individual learns of an innovation's existence; (b) *persuasion*–an individual forms a favorable or unfavorable attitude toward an innovation; (c) *decision*–an individual makes a decision to adopt or reject an innovation; (d) *implementation*–an individual puts the innovation to use; and (e) *confirmation*–an individual decides whether or not to use the innovation again.

Although the three processes described above have distinct characteristics, Oetting et al. (1995) note that they also share certain similarities: "They include the presence of a felt need, a period of information gathering, a stage of considering alternatives and developing plans, some form of initial implementation, and a commitment to continue beyond the initial adoption period" (p. 665). Despite the utility of these models as a useful point of departure for developing a model of community readiness, they proved inadequate in describing several key community processes, which include defining a local problem, deciding whether or not to take action, and considering the modification or expansion of existing programs (Donnermeyer et al., 1997). To more accurately portray these aspects, a revised model of the stages of community readiness was produced, which incorporated elements of psychological readiness for treatment and community development processes along with the experiences of prevention program practitioners and researchers (Donnermeyer et al., 1997; Oetting et al., 1995).

The resulting model of community readiness assesses communities along six dimensions and results in assigning the community to one of nine stages (Plested et al., 1998; Donnermeyer et al., 1997; Oetting et al., 1995). The six dimensions are: (a) community efforts such as programs, activities, and policies; (b) community knowledge of the efforts; (c) leadership, including appointed leaders and influential community members; (d) community climate; (e) community knowledge about the issue; and (f) resources related to the issue, such as people, money, time, and space.

The nine resulting stages are: (a) *no awareness*–the issue is not recognized by the community or its leaders as a problem; (b) *denial*–the community feels that the problem does not exist, or that change is impossible; (c) *vague awareness*–there is recognition of the problem, but not motivation for action; (d) *preplanning*–there is recognition of a problem and agreement that something needs to be done; (e) *preparation*–active planning is occurring; (f) *initiation*–a program has been implemented; (g) *stabilization*–one or two programs are operating and are stable; (h) *confirmation/expansion*–there is recognition of limitations and attempts to improve existing programs; and (i) *professionalization*–prevention efforts are marked by sophistication, training, and effective evaluation. With each successive stage in the community readiness model, there is corresponding improvement in the characteristics that promote community readiness.

The model of community readiness has promising practical utility. By interviewing key informants within each community (i.e., members of the community who are knowledgeable about prevention programs and have linkages with various community representatives), information is available to assess communities with regard to their readiness for a specific prevention program (for a thorough description of this process, refer to Donnermeyer et al., 1997; and Oetting et al., 1995). This assessment can then be used to (a) assign the community to a stage of readiness; (b) determine the likelihood of a program's effectiveness; (c) provide information on how finite resources can be allocated; and (d) develop and implement strategies to increase or improve community readiness (cf. Kumpfer et al., 1997). Increasing community readiness contributes to both the effectiveness and the continuity of prevention programs. Effective programs are more likely to be comprehensive, sustainable, well-planned, and coordinated at the local level (Kumpfer et al., 1997). These qualities, in turn, can significantly impact the modification of community norms and values. Prevention programs are more likely to achieve continuity when community members are involved and the program is responsive to the community's needs and resources. When efforts are sustained and longstanding, positive program impact and program outcomes can be realized. To the extent that it can encourage the development of these qualities, the community readiness model may serve as a useful tool in guiding prevention efforts.

The community readiness model offers promise to interventions that wish to establish different methods to conceptualize the communities they work with, and to inform ongoing interaction to progress toward intervention goals. This model offers users a unique perspective from which to observe the complex and dynamic ways in which communities and interventions interact. In this study, the model is adapted and applied to an intervention aimed at reducing youth access to tobacco.

SMOKING PREVENTION

Researchers have long grappled with the problem of reducing tobacco use as a way of optimizing the health and well-being of communities (Rhodes & Jason, 1988). From the early to the mid 1990s, current smoking, defined as having smoked in the past 30 days, increased from 27.8% to 34% for high school students, and increased from 15.5% to 21% for eighth graders (Johnston, 1996). Even though rates have begun to decrease 1 to 3 percentage points in the last two years, rates of smoking among American teens remain very high (Johnston, O'Malley, & Bachman, 1998). Each day, 3,000 American adolescents become established smokers (Gilpin, Choi, Berry, & Pierce, 1999), and it is estimated that 1,000 of these children will eventually die of tobacco related illnesses (Centers for Disease Control, 1996). Smoking is the leading preventable cause of death in the United States, killing over 400,000 people each year (Centers for Disease Control, 1993). Despite these facts, 22.9% of adult Americans and 13.8% of Americans under the age of 18 smoke cigarettes (Centers for Disease Control, 1996).

Nicotine addiction typically begins in adolescence with experimental cigarette smoking that progresses to smoking as a social activity and finally to regular, daily cigarette smoking. One of the risk factors for adolescent cigarette smoking is easy access to tobacco products (DiFranza, Carlson, & Caisse, 1992; Jason, Ji, Anes, & Birkhead, 1991; Stanton, Mahalski, McGee, & Silva, 1993). In the US, research conducted in the 1980s up to the mid 1990s found that in most areas minors could purchase cigarettes from retailers most of the time (Biglan et al., 1995; Jason, Ji, Anes, & Xaverious, 1992; Forster, Komro, & Wolfson, 1996; Johnston, 1995). Findings also indicate that adults in the US overwhelmingly support policies that limit minors' access to tobacco (Strouse & Hall, 1994). Although fewer vendors currently are selling minors cigarettes, youth still have easy access to tobacco products (Jason, Berk, Schnopp-Wyatt, & Talbot, 1999).

For over 12 years, a research group at DePaul University has been investigating methods of reducing youth access to tobacco at a community level (Jason et al., 1991; Jason et al., 1999). The current project is the Youth Tobacco Access Project (YTAP), which is a three-year project funded by The Robert Wood Johnson Foundation. YTAP is a randomized trial, multi-community intervention designed to examine the effectiveness of both sales and possession enforcement strategies to reduce youth access to tobacco. Communities were randomly assigned to experimental (sales and possession enforcement) or control (sales enforcement only) conditions. The study hypothesizes that the rate of tobacco use by youth in the experimental (i.e., sales and possession enforcement) condition will be significantly lower than in the control (i.e., sales enforcement only) condition. Across both experimental and control communities, the project assumes an active intervention component by increasing community awareness of tobacco-related issues, encouraging relevant intra-community communication and collaboration, providing communities with local data on youth tobacco use and tobacco merchant sales rates, and promoting the effectiveness of tobacco sales enforcements in reducing youth access to tobacco. It is hoped that the results of this study serve to inform public policy concerning the most effective strategies to reduce the use of tobacco by youth.

Because YTAP works with a number of systems within each community to achieve the intervention's goals, the project staff has developed linkages with schools, police, local health departments, and various community coalitions interested in reducing youth tobacco use. The opportunity to work with these multiple systems across eleven communities provides a unique vantage point from which to observe both the communities themselves, and the impact of the intervention. During the first year of this three-year project, the research team became interested in developing a method to keep track of the communities in relation to both the intervention's goals and to each other. It was easy to see that each community responded very differently to our presence, and each had unique characteristics that could influence the scope of the intervention. It became clear that a means to assess the communities on dimensions relevant to the intervention could serve a number of related purposes:

1. *Providing a Conceptual Heuristic*–Working with systems in multiple communities can be a harrowing task, particularly so when human resources are modest (i.e., the Youth Tobacco Access Project is staffed by three full-time employees). The opportunity to create categorical snapshots of each community could provide a framework for organizing a number of seemingly discrete community events and characteristics under a conceptual rubric. That rubric, in turn, could allow for a deeper understand-

ing of community-level dynamics, and allow for faster and more efficient processing of information relevant to interacting with each community throughout the intervention.

2. *Increasing Responsiveness*–The project attempts to employ an ecological perspective by demonstrating sensitivity to the needs of each community and by tailoring the intervention to their unique needs (Kelly, 1966; Kelly, 1968). The use of a system that would effectively and efficiently convey a community's status would facilitate responsiveness to factors in the intervention that compromised the intervention's progress.

3. *Measuring Changes Over Time*–Although extensive data were already being collected for the study, the opportunity to systematically measure the progress of each community for the duration of the intervention could provide information on each community's rate of adoption of intervention goals.

4. *Informing Strategies*–Perhaps the most important purpose of assessing communities in relation to the intervention is to provide a useful diagnostic system to inform community-specific strategies to increase the effectiveness of intervention efforts (Donnermeyer et al., 1997).

The community readiness model, with its focus on prevention programming and its roots in community development, appeared to provide the closest fit for our needs. By adopting the model to have a more behavioral focus, we hoped to establish the appropriate perspective and integrative framework from which to observe the communities participating in the intervention, and to contribute to the overall effectiveness of the intervention's efforts. Due to the specific nature of our intervention as one that examines strategies to reduce youth access to tobacco and potentially reduce the use of tobacco by youth, two scales of community readiness were selected for the current study: tobacco sales enforcements and tobacco possession enforcements. These scales are based upon research findings and hypotheses that indicate that each may play a critical role in reducing the use of tobacco by youth (cf. Cummings, 1997; cf. Lantz et al., 2000). Each scale consists of seven dimensions: (a) knowledge of the problem; (b) leadership; (c) resources; (d) community efforts; (e) knowledge of efforts; (f) town climate; and (g) police department climate. Although these dimensions may be related to each other, it is also possible that a community that is assessed at a high stage on one dimension may be assessed at a much lower stage on the others. Through the assessment of each dimension, we can ascertain the relative strengths and challenges present within each community. It was hypothesized that towns rated at higher stages of readiness would demonstrate higher levels of enforcement activity than towns rated at lower stages of readiness.

METHOD

Participants

Eleven towns in northern and central Illinois participated in the present study as a secondary activity of their participation in the primary intervention of the Youth Tobacco Access Project. Towns ranged in population from 9,401 to 107,001 ($M = 31,742$, $SD = 32,493$) and had a median household income between \$25,428 and \$60,979 ($M = \$34,924$, $SD = \$10,914$) (U.S. Census Bureau, 1990). The number of officers employed by each town's police department ranged from 8.0 officers per 10,000 residents to 45.9 officers per 10,000 residents ($M = 25.6$, $SD = 12.32$) (Harden Political InfoSystem, 2000) and the number of community police officers ranged from 0.5 officers per 10,000 residents to 39.8 officers per 10,000 residents ($M = 6.5$, $SD = 11.5$) (U. S. Department of Justice, 2000).

Procedures

From January 1999 through July 1999 interviews were conducted with key informants (i.e., Chief of Police) from the police department in each of the eleven towns. Two independent raters rated each town on two separate scales: a sales enforcement scale and a possession enforcement scale. When the independent ratings were complete, the two raters met to share their scores, discuss their reasoning for each score, and to come to a consensus on each score. After a score was agreed upon for each of the seven dimensions on each scale, the scores for each scale were summed and averaged. The average for each scale was then used to determine what stage each town was in for sales enforcement and for possession enforcement.

Data Analyses

Community readiness scores for sales enforcement were compared with the number of local police department compliance checks conducted in 1999 using a bivariate correlation. Compliance checks are a procedure in which the police department employs a minor to attempt to purchase tobacco from a retailer and follows consequent illegal tobacco sales to the minor with either an official warning or penalties pursuant to local or state law. For the purposes of these analyses, the number of compliance checks was determined by the self-reported response to the question, "How many inspections did you conduct?"

Community readiness scores for possession enforcement were compared with the rate of citations issued in 1999 using a bivariate correlation. The rate of citations was calculated based on the number of citations issued proportionate to the population of the town under the age of 18 years.

RESULTS

Inter-rater reliability for each scale was calculated using a bivariate correlation. Reliabilities for individual dimensions of the scale for sales enforcement readiness ranged from $0.94, p < .01$ to $1.0, p < .01$. Overall, the correlation for the sales enforcement ratings was $0.97, p < .01$. Reliabilities for individual dimensions of the scale for possession enforcement readiness ranged from 0.57 to $0.99, p < .01$. Overall, the correlation for the possession enforcement ratings was $0.86, p < .01$. Inter-rater reliability was assessed based on the 2001 readiness ratings.

Community readiness scores for 1999 sales enforcement ranged from 1.57 to 6.85 ($M = 3.94, SD = 1.96$) and readiness scores for 1999 possession enforcement ranged from 1.71 to 5.86 ($M = 4.09, SD = 1.52$). The number of local police department sales compliance checks for each retailer ranged from 0 to 4 ($M = 1, SD = 1.4$) and the rate of possession enforcement ranged from 0 to 2.7 ($M = 1.04, SD = 0.96$). The correlation between the readiness score for sales enforcement and the number of sales compliance checks was $0.88, p < .01$. The correlation between the readiness score for possession enforcement and the rate of citations was $0.52, p > .05$.

DISCUSSION

In this study, communities were rated on their readiness to implement tobacco sales and tobacco possession enforcement programs. Using an adaptation of the Community Readiness model, towns were rated on two separate, behaviorally based scales. It was hypothesized that towns rated at higher stages of readiness would demonstrate higher levels of enforcement activity than towns rated at lower stages of readiness. A significant correlation was found between the sales enforcement rating and the number of sales compliance checks conducted by the local police department. The correlation between the possession enforcement rating and the rate of possession citations was not significant, but was in the expected direction with towns with higher ratings issuing more citations than towns with lower ratings.

The purpose of this study was to describe efforts to adapt a model of community readiness for prevention efforts to a specific intervention to reduce youth access to tobacco. In doing so, we hoped both to inform our intervention and to assess the extent to which the conceptual stages of the community readiness model can be adapted to novel intervention endeavors (cf. Donnermeyer, 1997, p. 82). It was hoped that the stages could provide a framework for understanding the dynamics within each community in relation to each dimension of community readiness assessed. It may not be effective for an intervention to expect communities at different stages to progress in similar ways and at a similar pace toward desirable goals. Stage assessments may allow an intervention to monitor whether a community is proceeding in a manner that corresponds with their level of readiness. When this is not the case, the intervention can act quickly to assist the community in getting back on track.

The most practical utility of using the community readiness model as applied to a specific intervention is to inform strategies to move communities to higher stages of readiness. Different strategies are necessary at different stages of readiness (Edwards et al., 2000). Increased awareness of a community's readiness can facilitate the selection of strategies that have a greater likelihood of being successful within that particular community. For example, one suburban town was rated at the "Denial" stage of readiness for tobacco sales enforcements. This community had a local tobacco sales law but did not conduct enforcements with tobacco merchants because tobacco use by youth was not perceived as a widespread problem nor as an important issue. In this community, it was important to raise awareness of the issue of youth access to tobacco as a local problem. By providing local data from school surveys, the research team sensitized the police department to the public health issues; and through informing the department of the opportunity to participate in a state program that funded tobacco sales compliance checks, the research team reinforced the role of the police in responding to youth access to tobacco. The research team assisted the department in applying for the state funded program and, consequently, the department began conducting tobacco sales compliance checks on a routine basis and took steps to strengthen enforcement of other aspects of their local tobacco control ordinance, including enforcing merchant licensing requirements. As a result, at the time of the second readiness assessment the department had progressed from "Denial" about sales enforcements to "Stabilization."

For communities that have already achieved higher stages, intervention strategies geared toward lower stages may not be effective. In a mid-sized town surrounded by a rural area, efforts to raise community awareness about youth access to tobacco and the role of police in response to the issue would not have been the most appropriate strategy because the community was already active in enforcing tobacco sales laws. In this community, police enforcement of sales laws was better helped by stabilizing the existing community efforts and publicizing community progress and future plans. For this town, efforts focused on providing press releases to increase local media coverage of law enforcement efforts to expand their compliance checks and providing retailer feedback letters to raise awareness among retailers of enforcement activities and to reinforce those retailers who refused sales to minors. These activities helped to draw additional support for community-driven efforts consonant with the intervention goals.

In addition to planning stage-applicable strategies, the community readiness ratings can also be used to measure community change over time. Comparisons of stage ratings for the eleven communities for 1999 and for 2001 reveal patterns of progress. One community in particular is an exemplar of how community readiness ratings can measure community change over time, as this town demonstrated change on both the sales enforcement and possession enforcement ratings.

This suburban community located in a large metropolitan area moved from an initial sales enforcement stage rating of "Denial" to a rating of "Stabilization." The progress was due in large part to the town's decision to apply for state funding to conduct sales compliance checks. As part of the grant they received, the police department was obligated to conduct three rounds of compliance checks annually. This level of activity substantially increased their ratings on all dimensions. Additionally, the department distributed retailer feedback letters provided by the research team, organized a retailer education meeting facilitated by the state funding agency, and distributed retailer education packets provided by the state funding agency. At the time of the 2001 rating, the town had applied for a renewal of the state-sponsored enforcement program and planned to continue compliance checks indefinitely.

This community also demonstrated progress on readiness for possession enforcement. The town's progress on possession readiness from an initial stage rating of "Denial" to a rating of "Preparation" was the result of the passage of a new local tobacco control ordinance that explicitly defined possession of tobacco by minors as a violation of the law. The passage of the ordinance was assisted by the research team who provided a model tobacco control ordinance that was adapted by the city attorney's office, met with the chief of police to discuss how the ordinance would benefit the department, and spoke at a city council meeting to educate council members on the importance of the new ordinance. At the time of the 2001 ratings, the town had finalized their procedures for issuing tickets, and it is anticipated that with the commencement of possession enforcement the town would soon be rated in the "Stabilization" stage.

These examples reinforce that the community readiness model offers promise to interventions that wish to establish different methods to conceptualize the communities they work with and to inform ongoing progress toward intervention goals. The current study attempts to adapt the original model of community readiness to a specific intervention with multiple communities. To do so, the authors modified the model to correspond with the intervention's goals and validated the stage assessments with behavioral outcome data. Through continued validation, ongoing refinements can be made to a model that offers users a unique perspective from which to observe the complex and dynamic ways in which communities and interventions interact.

REFERENCES

Beal, G. M. (1964). Social action: Instigated social change in large social systems. In J. H. Copp (Ed.), *Our changing rural society: Perspectives and trends* (pp. 233-264). Ames, Iowa: Iowa State University Press.

Biglan, A., Henderson, J., Humphrey, D., Yasui, M., Whisman, R., Black, C., & James, L. (1995). Mobilizing positive reinforcement to reduce youth access to tobacco. *Tobacco Control, 4,* 42-48.

Burgoyne, N. S., & Jason, L. A. (1991). Incorporating the ecological paradigm into behavioral preventive interventions. In P. R. Martin (Ed.), *Handbook of behavior therapy and psychological science: An integrative approach.* (pp. 457-472). New York, NY: Pergamon Press.

Butterfoss, F. D., Goodman, R. M., & Wandersman, A. H. (1996). Satisfaction, partici-
    pation, and planning. *Health Education Quarterly, 23*, 65-79.
Centers for Disease Control. (1993). Cigarette smoking–attributable mortality and
    years of life lost–United States, 1990. *Morbidity and Mortality Weekly Report, 42*,
    645-649.
Centers for Disease Control. (1996). *State Tobacco Control Highlights–1996* (CDC
    Publication No. 099-4895). Atlanta: National Center for Chronic Disease Preven-
    tion and Health Promotion, Office on Smoking and Health.
Chavis, D. M., & Wandersman, A. H. (1990). Sense of community in the urban envi-
    ronment: A catalyst for participation and community development. *American Jour-
    nal of Community Psychology, 18*, 55-81.
Cummings, K. M. (1997). Health policy and smoking and tobacco use. In D. S.
    Gochman (Ed.), *Handbook of health behavior research IV: Relevance for profes-
    sionals and issues for the future* (pp. 231-251). New York: Plenum Press.
DiFranza, J. R., Carlson, R., & Caisse, R. (1992). Reducing youth access to tobacco.
    Tobacco Control, 14, 58.
Donnermeyer, J. F., Plested, B. A., Edwards, R. W., Oetting, E. R., & Littlethunder, L.
    (1997). Community readiness and prevention programs. *Journal of the Community
    Development Society, 28*, 65-83.
Edwards, R. W., Jumper-Thurman, P., Plested, B. A., Oetting, E. R., & Swanson, L.
    (2000). Community readiness: Research to practice. *Journal of Community Psy-
    chology, 28*, 291-307.
Edwards, R. W., Jumper Thurman, P., Plested, B. A., Oetting, E. R., & Swanson, L.
    (1999). Community readiness theory: Roots and structure. Submitted in A.
    Wandersman (Chair), *Bridging the gap between science and research*. Symposium
    conducted by the Center for Substance Abuse Prevention in Washington, DC.
Forster, J. L., Komro, K. A., & Wolfson, M. (1996). Survey of city ordinances and lo-
    cal enforcement regarding commercial availability of tobacco to minors in Minne-
    sota, United States. *Tobacco Control, 5*, 46-51.
Fuqua, D. R., Newman, J. L., & Dickman, M. M. (1999). Barriers to effective assess-
    ment in organizational consultation. *Consulting Psychology Journal: Practice and
    Research, 51*, 14-23.
Gilpin, E. A., Choi, W. S., Berry, C., & Pierce, J. P. (1999). How many adolescents
    start smoking each day in the United States? *Journal of Adolescent Health, 25*,
    248-255.
Goodman, R. M., Wandersman, A. H., Chinman, M., Imm, P., & Morrissey, E. (1996).
    An ecological assessment of community-based intervention for prevention and
    health promotion. *American Journal of Community Psychology, 24*, 33-61.
Hallman, W. K., & Wandersman, A. H. (1992). Attribution of responsibility and indi-
    vidual and collective coping with environmental threats. *Journal of Social Issues,
    48*, 101-118.
Harden Political InfoSys. (2000). *Cities and Towns InfoSystem* [On-line]. Available:
    www.prudentialalamo.com/Community/HPI.htm.
Howard-Pitney, B. (1990). Community development is alive and well in community
    health promotion. *The Community Psychologist, 234*, 8-9.

Jason, L.A., Berk, M., Schnopp-Wyatt, D.L., & Talbot, B. (1999). Effects of enforcement of youth access laws on smoking prevalence. *American Journal of Community Psychology, 27*, 143-160.

Jason, L. A., Ji, P. Y., Anes, M., & Birkhead, S. H. (1991). Active enforcement of cigarette control laws in the prevention of cigarette sales to minors. *Journal of American Medical Association, 266*, 3159-3161.

Jason, L. A., Ji, P. Y., Anes, M., & Xaverious, P. (1992). Assessing cigarette sales rates to minors. *Evaluation and the Health Professions, 15*, 375-384.

Johnston, L.D. (1995). Smoking rates climb among American teenagers, who find smoking increasingly acceptable and seriously underestimate the risks. Ann Arbor: The University of Michigan News and Information Service.

Johnston, L.D. (1996). Cigarette smoking continues to rise among American teenagers in 1996. Ann Arbor, MI: The University of Michigan.

Johnston, L. D., O'Malley, P. M., & Bachman, J. G. (1998). Monitoring the future study, 1998. (www.isr.umich.edu/src/mtf).

Jumper Thurman, P., Plested, B. A., & Edwards, R. W. (1999). Community readiness: A model for community mobilization. Submitted in A. Wandersman (Chair), *Bridging the gap between science and research.* Symposium conducted by the Center for Substance Abuse Prevention in Washington, DC.

Jumper Thurman, P., Plested, B. A., & Edwards, R. W., Helm, H. M., & Oetting E. R. (in press). Community readiness: A promising model for community healing. Department of Justice Monograph, Editor D. Bigfoot.

Jumper Thurman, P., Plested, B. A., & Edwards, R. W., & Oetting E. R. (in press–1998). Using the community readiness model in native communities. CSAP monograph.

Kelly, J. G. (1966). Ecological constraints on mental health services. *American Psychologist, 21*, 535-539.

Kelly, J. G. (1968). Toward an ecological conception of preventive interventions. In J. W. Carter, Jr. (Ed.), Research contributions from psychology to community mental health (pp. 75-99). New York, NY: Behavioral Publications.

Kumpfer, K. L., Whiteside, H. O., Wandersman, A. H., & Cardenas, E. (1997). *Community readiness for drug abuse prevention: Issues, tips, and tools.* Rockville, MD: National Institute on Drug Abuse (NIH Pub. No. 97-4111).

Lantz, P. M., Jacobson, P. D., Warner, K. E., Wasserman, J., Pollack, H. A., Berson, J., & Ahlstrom, A. (2000). Investing in youth tobacco control: A review of smoking prevention and control strategies. *Tobacco Control, 9*, 47-63.

Levine, M. (1998). Prevention and community. *American Journal of Community Psychology, 26*, 189-206.

Oetting, E. R., Donnermeyer, J. F., Plested, B. A., Edwards, R. W., Kelly, K., & Beauvais, F. (1995). Assessing community readiness for prevention. *The International Journal of the Addictions, 30*, 659-683.

Plested, B. A., Jumper Thurman, P., Edwards, R. W., & Oetting, E. R. (1998). Community readiness: A tool for effective community-based prevention. *Prevention Researcher, 5*(2).

Plested, B. A., Smithman, D. M., Jumper Thurman, P., Oetting, E. R., & Edwards, R. W. (1999). Readiness for drug abuse prevention in rural minority communities. *Substance Use & Misuse, 34*, 521-544.

Prochaska, J. O., DiClemente, C. C., Norcross, J. C. (1992). In search of how people change: Applications to addictive behaviors. *American Psychologist, 47*, 1102-1114.

Puddifoot, J. E. (1995). Dimensions of community identity. *Journal of Community & Applied Social Psychology, 5*, 357-370.

Puddifoot, J. E. (1996). Some initial considerations in the measurement of community identity. *Journal of Community Psychology, 24*, 327-336.

Rhodes, J. E., & Jason, L. A. (1988). *Preventing substance abuse among children and adolescents.* New York: Pergamon Press.

Rogers, E. M. (1983). *Diffusion of innovations* (3rd ed.). New York: Free Press.

Schooler, C., & Flora, J. A. (1997). Contributions of health behavior research to community health promotion programs. In D. S. Gochman (Ed.), *Handbook of Health Behavior Research IV: Relevance for Professionals and Issues for the Future* (pp. 285-302). New York, NY: Plenum Press.

Stanton, W. R., Mahalski, P. A. McGee, R., & Silva, P. A. (1993). Reasons for smoking or not smoking in adolescence. *Addictive Behavior, 18*, 321-329.

Strouse, R., & Hall, J. (1994). *Robert Wood Johnson Foundation youth access survey: Results of a national household survey to assess public attitudes about policy alternatives for limiting minor's access to tobacco products* (26023): Mathematical Policy Research, Inc.

U. S. Census Bureau. (1990). *United State Census, 1990* [On-line]. Available: www.census.gov

U. S. Department of Justice. (2000). *Office of Community Oriented Policing Services Grantee Report* [On-line]. Available: www.usdoj.gov/cops/

An Assessment of the Relationship Between the Quality of School-Based Tobacco Prevention Programs and Youth Tobacco Use

Stephanie M. Townsend

University of Illinois at Chicago

Steven B. Pokorny
Leonard A. Jason

DePaul University

Carrie J. Curie

University of Kansas

Michael E. Schoeny

University of Illinois at Chicago

SUMMARY. This study presents data from an assessment of substance use prevention programs in 23 elementary and middle schools in north-

Address correspondence to: Stephanie M. Townsend, Psychology Department, The University of Illinois at Chicago, 1007 West Harrison, Chicago, IL 60607-7137.

The authors express appreciation for financial support provided by the Robert Wood Johnson Foundation and David Altman, the National Program Director, and Andrea Williams, the Deputy Director, of the Substance Abuse Policy Research Program.

[Haworth co-indexing entry note]: "An Assessment of the Relationship Between the Quality of School-Based Tobacco Prevention Programs and Youth Tobacco Use." Townsend, Stephanie M. et al. Co-published simultaneously in *Journal of Prevention & Intervention in the Community* (The Haworth Press, Inc.) Vol. 24, No. 1, 2002, pp. 47-61; and: *Preventing Youth Access to Tobacco* (ed: Leonard A. Jason, and Steven B. Pokorny) The Haworth Press, Inc., 2002, pp. 47-61. Single or multiple copies of this article are available for a fee from The Haworth Document Delivery Service [1-800-HAWORTH 9:00 a.m. - 5:00 p.m. (EST). E-mail address: getinfo@haworthpressinc.com].

47

ern and central Illinois. The quality of prevention programming was assessed based on program intensity, focus on tobacco, staff resources designated for prevention programs, and implementation of the Centers for Disease Control and Prevention recommendations for tobacco prevention. Data from these four dimensions were used to calculate a Quality Index Score. Multilevel logistic regression analysis was used to assess the relationship between individual level variables, school level variables and the outcomes of reported current tobacco use, intent to use tobacco in the coming year, and perceived efficacy of substance use prevention programs. No significant effects were found, indicating that exclusive use of even high quality school-based prevention programs may not be sufficient in changing youth behavior. However, school-based prevention programs may be an important component of a broader ecological approach that uses multiple, community-wide strategies to promote normative change. *[Article copies available for a fee from The Haworth Document Delivery Service: 1-800-HAWORTH. E-mail address: <getinfo@ haworthpressinc.com> Website: <http://www.HaworthPress.com> © 2002 by The Haworth Press, Inc. All rights reserved.]*

KEYWORDS. Schools, minors, tobacco, prevention programs

Recent population estimates indicate that each day in the United States 4,800 youth try smoking for the first time and almost 3,000 more become established smokers (Gilpin, Choi, Berry, & Pierce, 1999). Tobacco experimentation and regular use increases throughout the middle school and high school years. Upon entering middle school, very few students report having used cigarettes (American Legacy Foundation, 2000). However, by the ninth grade almost one-fourth of students and by twelfth grade more than one-third of students report having used cigarettes (American Legacy Foundation, 2000). A youth's decision of whether or not to use tobacco has serious health consequences. Smoking is the leading preventable cause of death in the United States, killing over 400,000 people each year (Centers for Disease Control and Prevention, 1993). In addition to direct health consequences, the use of tobacco can also put youth at risk for subsequent use of alcohol and other drugs (Kandel, 1989).

Schools can be an important setting for educating youth about healthy behavior and for establishing norms pertaining to those behaviors (Brink, Simons-Morton, Harvey, Parcel, & Tiernan, 1988; Rhodes &

Jason, 1988). A variety of school-based programs for preventing tobacco use have been implemented over the past decades (Lantz et al., 2000). During the 1960s and 1970s, efforts to prevent the initiation of tobacco, alcohol, and other drug use were frequently designed to scare youth, to provide information about drugs and related paraphernalia, to appeal to adolescent morality, or to improve youths' self-esteem (Donaldson et al., 1996). Smoking prevention programs used curricula that were mostly aimed at increasing student awareness of the harmful, long-term effects of cigarette smoking (Perry, Killen, Telch, Slinkard, & Danaher, 1980).

In the 1980s, substance use prevention programs shifted toward curricula based on social influences (Donaldson et al., 1996).The social influences model of prevention education emphasizes the social environment as a critical factor in tobacco use (Lantz et al., 2000) and attempts to address environmental, personality and behavioral risk factors (Perry & Kelder, 1992). Tobacco prevention curricula based on the social influences model generally include seven major components: identification of short-term and long-term social consequences of use, reasons for tobacco use, information on peer norms, analysis of messages from media and role models, refusal skills, and public commitment activities (Perry & Kelder, 1992).

Despite four decades of studies on the effects of prevention programs on smoking rates among youth, there are no readily available tools for assessing the quality of substance use prevention programs in general or tobacco use prevention programs in particular. The evaluation tools that are available focus more on implementation strategies than on curriculum content and are often void of any specific recommendations regarding program content or delivery. Five aspects of school-based tobacco use prevention programs that may be important include use of an empirically based curriculum (Brounstein & Zweig, 1999), program intensity (Tobler, 1986; Tobler & Stratton, 1997), focus on tobacco (Johnson, MacKinnon & Pentz, 1996; Tobler & Stratton, 1997), staff resources (Bosworth, 1998), and adoption of guidelines for best practices published by the Centers for Disease Control and Prevention (CDC, 1994). Each of these aspects is discussed below.

The use of an empirically based curriculum can meet the demands of fiscal accountability that require substance use prevention programs to be validated (Tobler & Stratton, 1997). The Center for Substance Abuse Prevention (CSAP) defines science-based prevention programs as those that have been shown through research to be effective in the prevention or delay of substance use (Brounstein & Zweig, 1999). According to the

CSAP typology, empirically based curricula have minimally been subjected to an expert or peer consensus process or have appeared in a peer-reviewed journal. At the highest level are programs that have been replicated across populations and settings and appeared in several refereed professional journals. However, a survey of 104 school districts in 12 states and the District of Columbia found that the most widely used curricula are ones that have little or no empirically based research to show that they are effective in reducing substance use (Hallfors, Sporer, Pankratz & Godette, 2000).

Little research has been published concerning the effect of program intensity on the prevalence of substance use. In a meta-analysis of substance use prevention programs, Tobler and Stratton (1997) addressed the question of whether more intense programs, measured by hours of instruction, had greater positive effects. They found no significant effect due to program intensity. However, the lack of effect may be related to the fact that the mean intensity for all programs was only 10 hours. The high intensity programs were slightly more effective when instruction time was 18 hours. It is also possible that other factors such as the quality of the program itself may have affected these results. An earlier meta-analysis (Tobler, 1986) found a relationship between program intensity and effect size when accounting for the type of curriculum and mode of implementation. Poor quality programs, even when delivered with high intensity, may not produce the intended effect. Conversely, high quality programs that lack sufficient intensity may not yield significant effects.

The most widely used substance use prevention programs address a variety of substances, including tobacco, alcohol, and illegal drugs (Johnson et al., 1996). In considering whether it is more effective to target a single substance, multiple substances, or a broad range of lifestyle behaviors, Johnson et al. (1996) conducted a qualitative review of 13 studies. The programs studied differed primarily in whether the program focused exclusively on tobacco use, more broadly on tobacco, alcohol, and other drugs, or on healthy lifestyles that included prevention of tobacco, alcohol, and other drug use. The review found that multiple-purpose programs appeared no less effective for prevention of cigarette smoking than were programs that focused exclusively on tobacco use prevention. However, there is little corroboration for this conclusion and no tests for statistical significance were conducted. Therefore, specific instruction aimed at tobacco prevention may still be a factor in considering the effects of prevention programs on youth tobacco use.

Adequate staff resources to implement prevention efforts may also be important. A survey of 76 elementary, middle, and high schools found patterns of staff involvement in the development and implementation of substance use prevention curricula that indicate little use of resources outside of the local school (Bosworth, 1998). Of the schools surveyed, health teachers had the primary role in the development and implementation of substance use prevention curricula. The drug-free schools' coordinators were included in curriculum development in only 18% of schools and only 3% of schools used outside experts in the community. While the survey included only schools that developed their own prevention curricula rather than using commercially available curricula, it raises general questions about the use of staff resources at the school, district, and community levels. Schools, districts, or communities that allocate more resources to substance use prevention in the schools may have a stronger commitment and concern for the health of their youth.

Finally, adherence to the CDC's *Guidelines for School Health Programs to Prevent Tobacco Use and Addiction* should be considered (CDC, 1994). The guidelines represent expert opinions about best practices for tobacco use prevention and consist of seven recommendations. (A) Schools should have a comprehensive policy on tobacco. (B) The content of prevention instruction should include components equivalent to the social influences model of prevention. (C) Tobacco-use prevention education should be provided in each grade from kindergarten through grade 12. (D) Facilitators should receive program-specific training. (E) Parents and families should be involved in support of school-based prevention programs. (F) Schools should support cessation efforts among students and staff who use tobacco. (G) Prevention programs should be assessed at regular intervals to assess whether or not they are consistent with the CDC guidelines.

The present study is a secondary activity of the Youth Tobacco Access Project (Jason, Engstrom, Pokorny, Tegart, & Curie, 2000; Jason, Pokorny, Curie, Townsend, & Engstrom, 2002). The project is a three-year study designed to examine the impact of tobacco control policies on the prevalence of tobacco use among sixth, seventh, and eighth grade students in eleven communities in northern and central Illinois. In taking an ecological approach, it was determined that influences other than tobacco-control policies should be examined for potential effects on the prevalence rates of tobacco use. One potentially important influence identified was substance use prevention programs in the schools and an index for assessing the quality of school-based tobacco use prevention programs was developed. The quality of prevention programming was analyzed in relation to outcomes from a survey of sixth, seventh, and eighth grade students in the participating schools. Outcomes analyzed were students' current use of tobacco, intent to use tobacco in the coming year, and perceived efficacy of substance use prevention programs. It was hypothesized that students in schools with higher quality prevention programs would report lower amounts of current tobacco use, lower intent to use tobacco in the coming year, and higher perceived efficacy of substance use prevention programs.

METHOD

Participants

Twenty-three schools in northern and central Illinois participated in the present study. While the study focused on prevention education in the sixth, seventh, and eighth grades, the schools represented a variety of grade structures. Eight schools contained kindergarten through grade six, five schools contained kindergarten through grade eight, seven schools contained grades six through eight, and three schools contained grades seven and eight. A total of 5,992 students was surveyed. The racial background of students surveyed was 72.9% White (n = 4,374), 8.1% Latino (n = 487), 6.0% African American (n = 362), 5.2% multiracial (n = 314), 3.7% Asian/Pacific Islander (n = 220), 2.2% other (n = 133), 0.7% Middle Eastern (n = 43), and 0.4% Native American (n = 24). Thirty-five students (0.6%) did not identify their racial background. This racial distribution deviates in some categories from the demographics of the state of Illinois, which in 2000 reported a population under 18 years of age that was 66.8% White, 17% Latino, 18.7% African American, 3.0% multiracial, 3.0% Asian/Pacific Islander, 8.0% other, and 0.2% Native American (U. S. Census Bureau, 2001). Differences in racial distribution may be the result of the demographics of individual towns and/or generational differences in how youth versus their parents/guardians choose to identify race. The racial identity of youths who participated in the survey were comparable to the racial demographics of the towns in which the schools were located. The percentage of students coming from low-income families, as determined by eligibility for federal assistance programs in the schools and as based on total school population, ranged from 0.2% to 71.6% with a mean of 30.1% (Illinois State Board of Education, 2000).

Procedures

Prevention Programming Data. Data on tobacco use prevention education was collected in two phases. The first phase was comprised of a 45-item written survey that was self-administered by one key informant for each school. Key informants were identified by school personnel as the person primarily responsible for substance use prevention programs at the school. The key informant was an employee of the school, school district, a local governmental agency (i.e., police department or county health department), or a community services agency. The majority of questions on the survey were closed-ended and dichotomous and included questions about the grades targeted; amount of instructional time; amount of instructional time focused on tobacco, alcohol, and other drugs; adoption of CDC guidelines for tobacco use education; and program content.

The second phase consisted of a semi-structured interview with the key informant to clarify incomplete and ambiguous answers. In some cases the key informant was unable to provide information pertaining to certain aspects of the prevention program and the interviewer was referred to a secondary informant. Secondary informants were only questioned about the specific items the key informant could not answer.

Data collected from the written survey and follow-up interviews with key and secondary informants focused on five program-related variables pertaining to the 1999-2000 school year. (A) Program intensity was measured in hours of substance use prevention instruction provided in each grade per school year. (B) Focus on tobacco was measured in estimated hours per school year of substance use prevention instruction that were focused on tobacco use prevention. (C) Staff resources were determined based on the number of hours per school year the staff person(s) allocated to substance use prevention programming. (D) The CDC recommendations were developed into seven subscales, each having a total of 10 points possible. Each recommendation was divided into components (e.g., the recommendation concerning tobacco instruction was divided into five components: instruction on short-term effects, long-term effects, social norms, social influences, and refusal skills). Within each subscale, the components were given equal values. Prevention programs were evaluated on each subscale and the points were summed for a composite score. (E) Programs were identified as either empirically based or non-empirically based. The Western Regional Center for the Application of Prevention Technologies (WestCAPT) maintains a list of best practices for substance use prevention

(WestCAPT, 2000). Programs considered best practices are those that qualify as Type 3, Type 4, or Type 5 in the CSAP typology. For the purposes of this study, if a school's substance use prevention program appeared on the WestCAPT list of best practices, it was coded as an empirical curriculum. Programs that did not appear on the list were coded as non-empirical curricula.

All five programming variables were converted to standard scores to control for the wide range in data and were submitted to an analysis of bivariate correlation (see Table 1). Due to the high degree of correlation between average prevention instruction, average tobacco instruction, total staff resources, and the CDC subscales, these standard scores were summed to obtain a single Quality Index Score. Whether or not the school used an empirical curriculum was not significantly correlated with the other variables. While this variable may represent an important independent source of information, it was eliminated from the Quality Index Score due to the fact that only 2 out of 23 schools reported using an empirical curriculum, and therefore use of this variable did not allow for a clear assessment of the influence an empirical curriculum may have on the outcomes.

Student Data. Student data were collected from the annual student survey conducted by the Youth Tobacco Access Project. The survey of sixth, seventh, and eighth grade students in participating towns was completed in March and April of 2000 in the 23 participating schools. The survey consisted of 79 items and assessed demographic information, past and current use of specific tobacco products, behaviors related to obtaining tobacco products, knowledge of and attitudes about tobacco control policies, and past and current use of alcohol and other drugs by specific type of drug. To enhance the quality of the data, project staff administered the survey to students using standardized proce-

TABLE 1. Correlations of Quality Index Variables

	Prevention Instruction	Tobacco Instruction	Staff Resources	CDC	Empirical
Prevention Instruction		0.89**	0.70**	0.48*	−0.11
Tobacco Instruction	0.89**		0.48*	0.60**	0.66
Staff Resources	0.70**	0.48*		0.34	−0.08
CDC	0.48*	0.60**	0.34		0.48*
Empirical	−0.11	0.06	−0.08	0.48*	

*$p < 0.05$
**$p < 0.01$

dures. The participation rate was 84% (n = 5,992) of the enrolled 7,138 students.

For this assessment of prevention program effects, student level demographic variables were age, gender, grade, ethnicity, and presence of an adult tobacco user in the student's home. Age and grade were treated as continuous variables. Gender, ethnicity (White vs. minority) and presence of an adult tobacco user in the student's home were treated as dichotomous variables. Student level behavioral and attitudinal variables were students' current use of tobacco (i.e., in the past 30 days), intent to use tobacco within the next year, and perceived efficacy of school-based substance use education and prevention activities. Current tobacco use was a continuous variable that reflected the number of days tobacco was used in the past 30 days. Intent to use tobacco in the coming year was a dichotomous variable measured by students' yes/no responses to the question, "Do you think that you will be using tobacco products (like cigarettes, cigars, chewing tobacco, or snuff) a year from now?" Perceived efficacy of school-based substance use prevention programs was measured by students' responses on a five-point scale to the statement, "People under the age of 18 will smoke less because of the tobacco, alcohol, and other drug education and prevention activities in schools." Student responses were recoded to three levels: strongly disagree/disagree, neutral, and agree/strongly agree.

School level variables were school, school type, mobility rate, and the Quality Index Score. School type was included because tobacco use increases significantly by age (American Legacy Foundation, 2000), and since the prevention programs were implemented at schools with different grade structures it can be assumed that school type has a linear relationship to the outcomes of student behavior. Schools were coded as kindergarten through sixth grade; kindergarten through eighth grade or sixth through eighth grade; and seventh through eighth grade. School mobility rates were included due to suggestions that program effectiveness may be restricted for programs with high attrition rates (Tobler & Stratton, 1997). Mobility rates, defined as the sum of students transferring out of the school and students transferring into the school, divided by average daily enrollment, were obtained from the Illinois State Board of Education (ISBE) (ISBE, 2000) and were coded into two levels: low mobility (0–0.14) and high mobility (0.15 and higher).

Data Analyses

Data for one school (n = 251) were omitted due to an incomplete key informant survey and follow-up interview. The remaining data were analyzed using a multilevel, logistic regression model. Multilevel analysis was deemed a more precise analytic technique than a multivariate analysis of variance, as it accounts for the fact that implementation of prevention programs occurs at a group level, although the goal is to influence individual behavior (Kreft, 1998). The dependency of individual behavior on school level prevention programs must be accounted for in the analysis. Snijders and Bosker (1999) suggest that individual behavior may result from students sharing the same school environment, students sharing the same teachers, students within a school affecting each other by direct communication or shared group norms, and students coming from the same neighborhood. Multilevel analysis will correct for intraclass correlation, making it possible to estimate individual, group-level, and program effects (Kreft, 1998).

RESULTS

The average substance use prevention instruction in grades six through eight ranged from 0 hours to 60 hours ($M = 9.9$ hours, $SD = 14.2$) and the average focus on tobacco in grades six through eight ranged from 0 hours to 16 hours ($M = 2.6$ hours, $SD = 3.5$). Staff resources dedicated to substance use prevention ranged from 0 hours to 1,560 hours ($M = 290.1$ hours, $SD = 513$). Compliance with CDC recommendations as measured by a sum of seven subscales ranged from 3.75 to 48.65 out of a possible total of 70 ($M = 28.89, SD = 13.05$). Quality Index Scores ranged from -3.91 through 11.11 ($M = 1.69, SD = 4.03$). Mobility rates ranged from 0.02 through 0.59 ($M = 0.12, SD = 0.08$) (see Table 2).

Analyses conducted using a series of univariate, multilevel, logistic regression analyses identified no significant effects of school, school type, mobility rate, or Quality Index Score on current tobacco use, intent to use tobacco, or perceived efficacy of school-based substance use prevention programs. Due to the lack of significance in the univariate analyses, no analyses were conducted on possible interactive effects.

TABLE 2. Descriptive Statistics for Program Variables (N = 22 schools)

Variable	Minimum	Maximum	Mean	Std. Deviation
Average Prevention Instruction (hours)	0.00	60.00	9.90	14.20
Average Instruction on Tobacco (hours)	0.00	16.00	2.60	3.50
Total Staff Resources (hours)	0.00	1,560.00	290.10	513.60
CDC Subscales (sum)	3.75	48.65	28.89	13.05
Quality Index Score	−3.91	11.11	1.69	4.03
School Mobility Rate	0.02	0.59	0.12	0.08

DISCUSSION

In this study, the quality of substance use prevention programs was based on an assessment of program intensity, focus on tobacco, staff resources designated for prevention programs, and implementation of the CDC recommendations for tobacco prevention. Data in each of these categories were used to calculate a Quality Index Score. It was hypothesized that students in schools with higher Quality Index Scores would report lower amounts of current tobacco use, less intent to use tobacco in the future, and higher perceived efficacy of substance use prevention programs. When using multilevel logistic regression, the Quality Index Score was not significantly related to the outcomes of current use of tobacco (i.e., in the past 30 days), intent to use tobacco within the next year, and perceived efficacy of school-based substance use education and prevention activities.

These findings are consistent with one of the better controlled studies using the social influence approach that has recently generated considerable media attention. The Hutchinson Smoking Prevention Project (HSPP) (Peterson, Kealey, Mann, Marek & Sarason, 2000) was a 15 year randomized, controlled trial of smoking prevention among youth that provided a comprehensive social-influence intervention from grades three through twelve and assessed participants two years after high school graduation. HSPP findings on the prevalence of daily smoking for students indicated that there were no significant differences between students in the control and experimental conditions. However, there are several limitations in Peterson's study.

The number of prevention instruction hours in the Peterson study averaged 6.6 hours per year in grades 3 through 10. This level of prevention instruction does not meet the CDC recommendation of tobacco prevention instruction each year in grades kindergarten through 12 and is less than the instruction level of 18 hours at which Tobler and Stratton (1997) found greater program effects for general substance use prevention programs. Additionally, the study exerted no restrictions on prevention programs in the control group schools, thereby allowing for the possibility that some of the control schools may have also been using a social influences model program. This study does suggest, however, that caution needs to be used when drawing conclusions about the long-term effects of these types of person-oriented interventions.

Findings from the current study might suggest that tobacco prevention programs need to go beyond individual-oriented variables, and perhaps include distal influences, such as parental behavior, school policies, and community norms (Flay, 2000). Therefore, school-based tobacco prevention programs might be more effective when coordinated with multi-component, community strategies that attempt to reduce youth substance use. In other words, preventive interventions that focus exclusively on youth in school settings might overlook pernicious community influences on the initiation and maintenance of tobacco, alcohol, and other drug use. Interventions that rely exclusively on school-based curricula may have a small effect on student behavior, and community influences might need to be considered (Jason, Biglan, & Katz, 1998). Prevention programs that are most effective might involve multiple dimensions including media advocacy, youth anti-tobacco activities, family communications about tobacco use, reducing youth access to tobacco media, and comprehensive school programs (Biglan et al., 1996; Flay et al., 1994; Kaufman, Jason, Sawlski, & Halpert, 1994; Pechmann, 1997; Perry & Kelder, 1992).

This study indicates that an assessment of the quality of tobacco prevention instruction in schools is not related to effects of such prevention programs. However, school-based prevention programs may be an important component of a broader ecological approach. Further research is needed to examine the interactive effects of multiple, coordinated, community-wide strategies such as media campaigns, policy interventions to reduce youth access to tobacco, increased excise taxes on tobacco, and empirically based prevention programs in the schools that include family involvement. The coordinated implementation of strategies such as these may result in normative change within a community that promotes tobacco-free behavior by youth.

REFERENCES

American Legacy Foundation. (2000). *Cigarette smoking among youth: Results from the 1999 National Youth Tobacco Survey* (Legacy First Look Report). Washington, DC: American Legacy Foundation.

Biglan, A., Ary, D. V., Yudelson, H., Duncan, T. E., Hood, D., James, L., Koehn, V., Wright, Z., Black, C., Levings, D., Smith, S., & Gaiser, E. (1996). Experimental evaluation of a modular approach to mobilizing antitobacco influences of peers and parents. *American Journal of Community Psychology, 24* (3), 311-339.

Bosworth, K. (1998). Assessment of drug abuse prevention curricula developed at the local level. *Journal of Drug Education, 28,* 307-325.

Brink, S. G., Simons-Morton, D. G., Harvey, C. M., Parcel, G. S., & Tiernan, K. M. (1988). Developing comprehensive smoking control program in schools. *Journal of School Health, 58,* 177-180.

Brounstein, P. J., & Zweig, J. M. (1999). Toward the 21st century: A primer on effective programs. *Monographs of the U. S. Department of Health and Human Services,* (DHHS Publication No. [SMA] 99-3301).

Centers for Disease Control and Prevention. (1993). *Cigarette smoking–attributable mortality and years of life lost–United States, 1990.* (Morbidity and Mortality Weekly Report No. 42). Atlanta, Georgia: U. S. Department of Health and Human Services.

Centers for Disease Control and Prevention. (1994). *Guidelines for school health programs to prevent tobacco use and addiction.* (Morbidity and Mortality Weekly Report No. 43). Atlanta, Georgia: U. S. Department of Health and Human Services.

Donaldson, S. I., Sussman, S. M., Mackinnon, D. P., Severson, H. H., Glynn, T., Murray, D. M., & Stone, E. J. (1996). Drug abuse prevention programming. *American Behavioral Scientist, 39,* 868-883.

Flay, B. R. (2000). Approaches to substance use prevention utilizing school curriculum plus social environment change. *Addictive Behaviors, 27,* 861-885.

Flay, B. R., Hu, B., Siddiqui, O., Day, L. E., Hedeker, D., Petraitis, J., Richardson, J., & Sussman, S. (1994). Differential influence of parental smoking and friends' smoking on adolescent initiation of smoking and escalation of smoking. *The Journal of Health and Social Behavior, 35,* 248-265.

Gilpin, E. A., Choi, W. S., Berry, C., & Pierce, J. P. (1999). How many adolescents start smoking each day in the United States? *Journal of Adolescent Health, 25,* 248-255.

Hallfors, D., Sporer, A., Pankratz, M., & Godette, D. (2000). Drug free schools survey: Report of results. (Report to The Robert Wood Johnson Foundation). Chapel Hill, NC: University of North Carolina at Chapel Hill.

Illinois State Board of Education. (2000). *School Report Cards* [On-line]. Available: <http://206.166.105.128/ReportCard/rchome.asp>.

Jason, L. A., Biglan, A., & Katz, R. (1998). Implications of the tobacco settlement for the prevention of teenage smoking. *Children's Services: Social Policy, Research, and Practice, 1*, 63-82.

Jason, L. A., Pokorny, S. B. Curie, C. J., Townsend, S. M., & Engstrom, M. (2002). Ecological Issues in Helping Communities Control Youth Access to Tobacco. Submitted for publication.

Jason, L. A., Engstrom, M. D., Pokorny, S. B., Tegart, G., & Curie, C. J. (2000). Putting the community back into prevention: Think locally, act globally. *Journal of Primary Prevention, 21*, 25-29.

Johnson, C. A., MacKinnon, D. P., & Pentz, M. A. (1996). Breadth of program and outcome effectiveness in drug abuse prevention. *American Behavioral Scientist, 39*, 884-896.

Kandel, D. B. (1989). Issues of sequencing of adolescent drug use and other problem behaviors. In B. Segal (Ed.), *Perspectives on Adolescent Drug Use* (pp. 55-76). New York: Haworth Press.

Kaufman, J. S., Jason, L. A., Sawlski, L. M., & Halpert, J. A. (1994). A comprehensive multi-media program to prevent smoking among black students. *Journal of Drug Education, 24*, 95-108.

Kreft, I. G. G. (1998). An illustration of item homogeneity scaling and multilevel analysis techniques in the evaluation of drug prevention programs. *Evaluation Review, 22*, 46-77.

Lantz, P. M., Jacobson, P. D., Warner, K. E., Wasserman, J., Pollack, H. A., Berson, J., & Ahlstrom, A. (2000). Investing in youth tobacco control: A review of smoking prevention and control strategies. *Tobacco Control, 9*, 47-63.

Pechmann, C. (1997). Do anti-smoking ads combat underage smoking? A review of past practices and research. In M. G. Goldberg, M. Fishbein, & S. Middlestadt (Eds.), *Social marketing: Theoretical and practical perspectives* (pp. 189-216). Hillsdale, NJ: Lawrence Erlbaum Associates.

Perry, C. L., & Kelder, S. H. (1992). Models for effective prevention. *Journal of Adolescent Health, 13*, 355-363.

Perry, C. L., Killen, J., Telch, M., Slinkard, L. A., & Danaher, B. G. (1980). Modifying smoking behavior of teenagers: A school-based intervention. *American Journal of Public Health, 70*, 722-725.

Peterson, A.V., Kealey, K. A., Mann, S. L., Marek, P. M., & Sarason, I.G. (2000). Hutchinson smoking prevention project: Long-term randomized trial in school-based tobacco use prevention–results on smoking. *Journal of the National Cancer Institute, 92*, 1979-1991.

Rhodes, J., & Jason, L. A. (1988). *Preventing substance abuse among adolescents.* New York: Pergamon.

Snijders, T., & Bosker, R. (1999). *Multilevel analysis: An introduction to basic and advanced multilevel modeling.* Thousand Oaks, CA: Sage Publications.

Tobler, N. S. (1986). Meta-analysis of 143 adolescent drug prevention programs: Quantitative outcome results of program participants compared to a control or comparison group. *Journal of Drug Issues, 16,* 537-567.

Tobler, N. S., & Stratton, H. H. (1997). Effectiveness of school-based drug prevention programs: A meta-analysis of the research. *Journal of Primary Prevention, 18,* 71-128.

U. S. Census Bureau. (2001). *United States Census, 2000* [On-line]. Available: <factfinder.census.gov>.

Western Regional Center for the Application of Prevention Technologies. (2000). *Alphabetical Listing of Best Practices* [On-line]. Available: <www.open.org/~westcapt/bpalpha.htm>.

An Examination of Factors Influencing Illegal Tobacco Sales to Minors

Carrie J. Curie

University of Kansas

Steven B. Pokorny
Leonard A. Jason

DePaul University

Michael E. Schoeny
Stephanie M. Townsend

University of Illinois at Chicago

SUMMARY. This study examined factors that influence illegal tobacco sales to minors, such as buyer, clerk, and store characteristics. Thirty-seven youths made 314 attempts to purchase tobacco in 11 towns in Illinois. Purchase attempts were made from over-the-counter and vending machine vendors. Multilevel multivariate logistic regression analyses, which controlled for town clustering effects, were run to determine predictors of illegal sales to minors. Findings revealed that the strongest pre-

---

Address correspondence to: Carrie J. Curie, Department of Human Development, University of Kansas, Lawrence, KS 66045.

The authors express appreciation for financial support provided by the Robert Wood Johnson Foundation and David Altman, the National Program Director, and Andrea Williams, the Deputy Director, of the Substance Abuse Policy Research Program.

[Haworth co-indexing entry note]: "An Examination of Factors Influencing Illegal Tobacco Sales to Minors." Curie, Carrie J. et al. Co-published simultaneously in *Journal of Prevention & Intervention in the Community* (The Haworth Press, Inc.) Vol. 24, No. 1, 2002, pp. 63-76; and: *Preventing Youth Access to Tobacco* (ed: Leonard A. Jason, and Steven B. Pokorny) The Haworth Press, Inc., 2002, pp. 63-76. Single or multiple copies of this article are available for a fee from The Haworth Document Delivery Service [1-800-HAWORTH 9:00 a.m. - 5:00 p.m. (EST). E-mail address: getinfo@haworthpressinc.com].

dictors of selling cigarettes illegally to minors were clerks' failure to ask a minor for age or identification. The implications of using multivariate methods to identify factors influencing illegal tobacco sales are discussed. *[Article copies available for a fee from The Haworth Document Delivery Service: 1-800-HAWORTH. E-mail address: <getinfo@haworthpressinc. com> Website: <http://www.HaworthPress.com> © 2002 by The Haworth Press, Inc. All rights reserved.]*

KEYWORDS. Tobacco, minors, illegal sales, merchants, youth access

Recent estimates indicate that each day 5,500 children try smoking for the first time, and almost 3,000 more become established smokers (Gilpin, Choi, Berry & Pierce, 1999). In the United States, first use of a tobacco product almost always occurs before high school graduation (Centers for Disease Control [CDC], 1994). Easy availability of tobacco products among youngsters might contribute to alarmingly high rates of tobacco use (Rhodes & Jason, 1988). Despite laws prohibiting the sale of tobacco products to persons under the age of 18, most minors have little difficulty purchasing cigarettes (Jason et al., 1999; Jason, Biglan, & Katz, 1998). It is unclear which minor, clerk, or store characteristics might influence youths' ability to purchase tobacco products illegally.

Previous research examining illegal tobacco sales to minors has suggested that a minor's ability to purchase tobacco may be influenced by specific buyer characteristics, such as the minor's age and/or gender. DiFranza, Savageau and Aisquith (1996), for example, found that youth who appeared to be 16 and 17 years of age were more successful in illegally purchasing tobacco than youth who appeared to be 11 to 15 years of age. O'Grady, Asbridge and Abernathy (1999) found that older minors were the most successful and the younger minors were least successful in illegally purchasing tobacco. Clark, Natanblut, Schmitt, Wolters and Iachan (2000) also found that the success rate in purchasing cigarettes increased with each increasing year of age. However, one study by Arday, Klevens, Nelson, Huang, Giovino and Mowrey (1997) did not find a relationship between apparent age and sales outcome.

When gender has been examined as a predictor of illegal sales, the literature suggests that girls are more frequently sold cigarettes. Arday et al. (1997), DiFranza et al. (1996), and Clark et al. (2000) found that girls were more successful than boys during the purchase attempts. When two minors conducted a purchase attempt together, O'Grady et al. (1999) found that mixed dyads (males and females) were the most successful when attempting to illegally purchase tobacco followed by female dyads, with male dyads being the least successful.

When exploring what type of clerk behavior is a predictor of sales outcome, asking a minor for age or identification substantially reduces illegal sales. Landrine, Klonoff, and Alcaraz (1997) found that when age or ID was requested, illegal sales were significantly less likely to occur. If minors were questioned by clerks about their age during a tobacco purchase attempt, 96% of the time they were refused cigarettes, and if the clerk requested identification from the minor, 99% of the time the tobacco sale was refused. Clark et al. (2000) also found a significant relationship between a clerk's request for proof of age and refusal of sales. Minors were refused illegal sales 90% of the time when asked for proof of age.

Several studies have examined the relationship between gender and being questioned about age or identification. Arday et al. (1997) noted that female buyers were less likely to be questioned by clerks during a tobacco purchase attempt. DiFranza et al. (1996), however, found that boys and girls were equally likely to be asked for proof of age. Landrine et al. (1996) also did not find gender differences with respect to questioning a minor during a purchase attempt. Only one researcher, to date, has examined the relationship between a field agent's ethnicity and being asked about age or identification. Landrine et al. (1996) found that African American youth were asked their age and ID significantly more than white youth.

Several studies have also examined whether a successful purchase attempt may be associated with clerk characteristics, such as the clerks' apparent age and/or gender. DiFranza et al. (1997) found that younger clerks (estimated to be under 21 years of age) were more likely to sell to minors than older clerks (estimated to be over 21 years of age). However, Arday et al. (1997) did not find the estimated clerks' age to be related to a successful sales outcome. Forster, Wolfson, Murray, Wagenaar and Claxton (1997) noted that male clerks had a tendency to sell more frequently to minors than female clerks. Contrary to those findings, Clark et al. (2000) found that female clerks were more likely to sell to underage youth. However, Arday et al. (1997) did not find the clerks' gender to be related to a successful sales outcome.

Along with individual characteristics that pertain to purchase success, researchers have examined whether store characteristics play a role in determining sales outcome. Forster et al. (1997) found that gas stations and convenience stores were most likely to sell cigarettes to youth followed by grocery stores and restaurants. Clark et al. (2000) found that gas stations had the highest sales rates, but convenient stores that did not sell gas had the lowest sales rates. However, Arday et al. (1997) found no relationship between type of store and successful sales outcome when looking only at stores with over the counter sales. O'Grady et al. (1999) also did not find a relationship between type of store and purchase success rates.

When examining the type of tobacco product access, Forster et al. (1997) found that when tobacco products are locked up or behind a counter accessible only to the clerk, they are less likely to sell tobacco to minors. In addition, youth tend to have more success purchasing tobacco products from vending machines that are unlocked than from vendors with over the counter sales (DiFranza et al., 1996).

Other variables that may relate to sales outcome are tobacco advertising and tobacco sales promotions (Wakefield et al., 2000). Several studies have evaluated whether vendor-warning signs relating to the laws prohibiting the sale of tobacco to minors may have some influence on sales outcome. DiFranza et al. (1996) found that stores that participated in "It's the Law" programs, which involved posting vendor-warning signs were somewhat more likely to request proof of age from minors attempting to illegally purchase tobacco, but the differences in questioning did not result in a reduction in illegal sales. Arday et al. (1997) found that warning signs had no effect on vendors' compliance with the state minors' access law. Although clerks in stores with warning signs posted were somewhat more likely to ask questions of the minor during the purchase attempt, stores with warning signs were actually associated with a higher likelihood of selling to minors. Forster et al. (1997) indicated that the presence of tobacco-industry or other signs that made a reference to tobacco sales law were not associated with purchase success.

Finally, the presence or absence of store customers at the time of the purchase attempt may play a role in determining sales outcome. Forster et al. (1997) examined the environment of the store at the time of the purchase attempt and found that the presence of one or more customers in line behind a youth buyer positively predicted purchase success.

Clearly, the literature reviewed above is mixed concerning the role of minor, clerk, and store characteristics that might influence illegal sales of cigarettes. Many of the studies reviewed above examined certain aspects of these characteristics, but rarely have the comprehensive array of various youth, clerk, and store characteristics been examined simultaneously using multifactorial analyses. It is possible that the discrepant findings reviewed above are due to past studies focusing on selective variables (i.e., minor characteristics only, clerk characteristics only, or store characteristics only). The purpose of this study was to examine multiple youth, clerk, and store influences that might affect illegal tobacco sales to minors.

METHODS

The data for the present study were obtained from an assessment of 314 retail tobacco sales attempts to minors within each of 11 towns in Illinois. Towns were selected based on a population of 5,000 or more individuals. The assessment of retail tobacco sales to minors involved identifying tobacco retailers, recruiting youth to be field agents, and training the youth to conduct tobacco purchase attempts. The data were collected in July and August of 1999.

Retail Tobacco Sales to Minors

Identification of Tobacco Retailers. A list of all licensed tobacco retailers was obtained from the City Clerk's Office in each town that had an ordinance requiring these merchants to be licensed. In towns that did not have an ordinance for licensing tobacco retailers, project staff used a standard protocol for identifying tobacco retailers. Project staff used an Internet based telephone directory available through "Yahoo.com" to identify all potential tobacco retailers located within the town limits. Specific directory categories of businesses likely to sell cigarettes (e.g., convenience stores, gas stations, restaurants, etc.) were searched in the Internet directory. To discover which retailers on the list actually sold tobacco products, a research assistant placed a carefully scripted telephone call to each retailer asking if they sold tobacco products. The scripts were phrased to ensure that the purpose of the call was not evident to the retailer.

The list of identified tobacco retailers was then given to a liaison from the local police department for further validation and editing. The police liaison was asked to check the list for any possible omissions and to eliminate any inappropriate retailers. Retailers were removed if they: (1) were no longer in business or no longer sold tobacco products, (2) were taverns or bars that serve liquor only (i.e., no food or primarily served liquor with a limited menu), (3) were adult-oriented businesses,

(4) were generally inappropriate for 15- and 16-year-old girls, or (5) were unavailable for assessment at the time of our Tobacco Purchase Attempts (e.g., retailers closed for the season and retailers not open at the time of the Tobacco Purchase Attempts). After completing the retailer identification and validation process described above, there were 314 appropriate retailers throughout the 11 towns.

Recruitment of Field Agents. In each town, the liaison from the police department was asked to recruit youth to participate as Field Agents for the Tobacco Purchase Attempts. In order to standardize our procedure across towns and minimize potential bias, only non-smoking female youth aged 15 or 16 were recruited as field agents for this project. Liaisons were supplied with recruitment materials, which included: (1) a project brochure to help describe the project to parents and youth, (2) consent forms for youth to participate as Field Agents in this study, (3) visual age assessment rating forms for rating the age appearance of potential Field Agents, and (4) a sample of a letter to provide the Field Agents with immunity from prosecution.

Three procedures that were essential to the recruitment process included the consent procedure, the age appearance rating, and the letter of immunity. Informed, active consent was necessary from both the youth and one of their parents/legal guardians in order for the youth to participate in the Tobacco Purchase Attempts. In addition, the liaison police officer was asked to confirm that participating youth actually looked 15 or 16 years old by obtaining two Visual Age Assessment Ratings for each youth. It was thought that due to the nature of police business, police officers had adequate training in identifying the age of perpetrators, thus they were asked to confirm the age of the youth. Finally, each youth participating in the project was provided with a letter of immunity from prosecution from the police department. The letter was written to insure that neither the youth nor the retailer would be prosecuted as a result of their actions in this study.

Field Agent Characteristics

Caucasian females (sixteen 15-year-olds, and eleven 16-year-olds) and non-White females (six 15-year-olds and four 16-year-olds) participated as field agents in the Tobacco Purchase Attempts across the eleven communities. Parental consent was obtained for all of the youth, and youth were paid $5 per hour. In addition, youth were asked to wear casual clothes (jeans and T-shirt/sweatshirt); and clothes that did not indicate police or school affiliation. They were also asked to wear clothes that did not display any tobacco or alcohol images, and to wear little or no makeup or jewelry.

Training of Field Agents. On the day of the scheduled Tobacco Purchase Attempts, project staff held a 90-minute training session for the recruited youth at the police station. Before the youth began the training, they were required to provide project staff with completed Parent Consent forms. The youth were also asked to sign the Child Assent forms, provide proof of age, and give project staff emergency contact information prior to the training. The police liaison provided project staff with the age assessment ratings completed by two independent judges.

The training was designed to: (1) provide a description of Tobacco Purchase Attempts, (2) inform youth of Field Agent guidelines and responsibilities, (3) teach Field Agents what to say and do while conducting a Tobacco Purchase Attempt, (4) provide a description of four possible types of Tobacco Purchase Attempts (i.e., locked vending machine sales, unlocked vending machine sales, over-the-counter sales, and self-service sales), (5) teach the information collection protocol to Field Agents, and (6) prepare Field Agents for the Tobacco Purchase Attempts using role playing techniques.

Tobacco Purchase Attempt Protocol. A standard protocol was utilized for completing the Tobacco Purchase Attempts (TPA). Field Agents were driven to all appropriate vendors by project staff. Field Agents entered establishments that sold tobacco products and made the purchase attempts. During the TPAs, project staff remained outside of the establishment in an unobtrusive location.

Field Agents were asked to enter the business and locate the tobacco (i.e., vending machine, self-service display, or over-the-counter). When there was a vending machine, the Field Agent attempted to purchase cigarettes directly from the vending machine, and she asked the clerk to unlock any vending machine that had a locking device. If no one stopped the Field Agent or questioned her age, she deposited the quarters in the machine and purchased a pack of cigarettes. When there was a self-service display of tobacco, the Field Agent selected the most popular brand of cigarettes in their town as instructed during the Field Agent training (e.g., Marlboro Red, Marlboro Lights, Newports in a box, etc.), and placed it on the cashier's counter with the money. When the tobacco was available as an over-the-counter purchase, the Field Agent requested the most popular brand of cigarettes in their town (e.g., Marlboro Red, Marlboro Lights, Newports in a box, etc.), and placed the money on the counter.

When asked for their age during any type of Tobacco Purchase Attempt, Field Agents responded by stating their true age. When asked for identification during any type of Tobacco Purchase Attempt, Field Agents stated, "I'm sorry, I don't have my ID with me." Field Agents were instructed to leave the location of a purchase attempt if they saw someone they knew (e.g., clerk or customer). When a Field Agent knew the clerk, an alternate Field Agent assessed the retailer later in the day. Field Agents were instructed to remain courteous during a Tobacco Purchase Attempt and keep conversation to a minimum. Field Agents were encouraged to express any concerns that they had regarding their safety (e.g., suspicious looking people in or near the store) and were instructed to abort the purchase attempt immediately if they felt unsure about their safety.

Although according to Illinois state law illegal for minors to purchase tobacco, the data collection protocol described above has been endorsed as legal by city and state officials and by the FDA when conducting these types of assessments for research purposes or for enforcements. Results from these assessments, however, were not used for enforcement. As mentioned earlier, a letter of immunity from prosecution was obtained from each police department to cover the youth serving as field agents, as well as the tobacco merchants.

Tobacco Purchase Attempt Data Collection

After each Tobacco Purchase Attempt, project staff immediately recorded all information reported by the Field Agent relating to various store characteristics.

Field Agent Characteristics. As mentioned before, the age and ethnicity of the Field Agents were recorded. Field Agents were classified as White or non-White. There were 27 White youth. Non-Whites included 7 African-Americans, 2 Asian-Americans, and 1 Latina.

Clerk Characteristics. To determine the approximate age of the clerk, Field Agents were asked to indicate if they thought the clerk was 20 years of age or under, or 21 years of age or older. Field Agents were also asked to report the gender of the clerk. The Field Agents were also questioned about whether the clerk asked for their age, or if the clerk asked the Field Agent to show some type of identification.

Store Characteristics. To assess general store characteristics, project staff observed and recorded several qualities of the retail establishment from the car. Type of store was categorized as: Convenience Store, Gas/Service Station, Recreation/Restaurant/Other, or Supermarket/Drug

Store/Department Store. Stores were dummy coded in the analyses so that each store type was compared to convenience stores as the reference group. Project staff also recorded whether the store was part of a local or national chain. Staff also recorded the amount of tobacco advertising on the front and outside grounds of each retailer. The number of industry tobacco signs (signs that were created by tobacco companies that carried advertising logos) and merchant tobacco signs (handmade or vendor generated signs) were recorded.

Field agents were then questioned about various characteristics of the store. The type of access to tobacco products that the merchant provided for customers (i.e., over the counter sales or vending machine sales) was recorded. The Field Agent was asked if they saw a warning sign posted about the law, how many customers there were standing in line behind them (if the tobacco purchase attempt was over-the-counter), whether there was a self-service display of tobacco, and if there were any tobacco promotions or deals near the counter (e.g., buy two get one free, buy one get a free lighter, etc.).

Outcome Measures

To determine if the sale was refused or permitted, or if the store clerk indicated they did not carry tobacco products, field agents were questioned when they returned to the car immediately after each attempt. If the sale was permitted, the pack of cigarettes and any left over change was turned over to project staff immediately and the cost of the cigarettes was recorded.

Statistical Analyses

Chi-square analyses were first used to examine univariate relations between predictor variables and sales outcome. Next, a multilevel, logistic regression model was used to examine the relation between the individual predictor variables and the sales outcome, controlling for the town effect. Towns were included in the model as random effects to control for possible clustering effects. Finally, those variables found to be significant in the univariate, multilevel, logistic regression were entered into a multivariate, multilevel, logistic regression model. The statistical package used for the multilevel analyses was MIXOR (Hedeker & Gibbons, 1996).

RESULTS

Table 1 presents the individual minor, clerk and store characteristics predictor variables, and the percent of clerks not selling minors cigarettes. Using chi-square analyses, and not controlling for town effects, asking for ID or age, over-the-counter sales, type of store, and younger field agent age were significant predictors of merchants not selling to minors.

When the influence of towns was controlled, using a series of univariate, multilevel, logistic regression analyses, only three of the five variables mentioned above were significant: asking for age, asking for identification, and over-the-counter vs. vending machine sales (see Table 1). When these three variables were included in the multivariate model, and random effects of towns were controlled for, asking for age and asking for ID were the only significant variables in preventing illegal tobacco sales (see Table 2).

DISCUSSION

The findings from the present study indicate that a clerk questioning a minor about age and identification are the most significant deterrents of illegal tobacco sales. When a clerk asked the minor for identification, 97.5% of the time clerks refused to sell minors cigarettes. When clerks requested the minor's age, sales were refused 93.2% of the time. These findings are consistent with research conducted by Arday et al. (1997), Landrine et al. (1997), and Clark et al. (2000).

During the first step of our statistical analytic process, five variables were related to merchants not selling minors cigarettes. These variables included not asking for age or ID, over-the-counter sales, younger Field Agent age, and certain types of settings. When we controlled for the town effects, three variables were no longer significant: type of store, field agent age, and over-the-counter sales. In general, these findings suggest that there is town variation in these measures, and when town variance is controlled, these variables are no longer significant. When we controlled for town effects and when we employed multivariate analyses, only two variables, asking for age or ID, remained significant. These findings suggest that some of the significant findings from prior investigations might no longer be significant influences after accounting for the variance explained by asking for age or ID.

TABLE 1. Univariate Predictor Variables

Variable	Sale Refused %	Chi-Square Analyses	Univariate Logistic Regression Analyses
Field Agent Characteristics			
Field Agent Age			
15	83.3	**	
16	64.2		
Field Agent Race			
White	78.1		
Non-White	67.4		
Clerk Characteristics			
Clerk asked for age			
Yes	93.2	**	**
No	72.2		
Clerk asked for ID			
Yes	97.5	**	**
No	34.8		
Age of the clerk			
Under 20	71.8		
21 and over	77.0		
Gender of the clerk			
Male	70.6		
Female	79.9		
Store Characteristics			
Type of Store			
Convenience	77.0	**	
Gas-Service Station	73.4		
Recreation/Other	60.0		
Restaurant	54.8		
Supermarket/Drug/Department Store	86.5		
Merchant is part of a local or national chain			
Yes	77.5		
No	71.4		

TABLE 1 (continued)

Variable	Sale Refused %	Chi-Square Analyses	Univariate Logistic Regression Analyses
Number of Industry signs present			
0	75.9		
1	63.8		
2	74.4		
3	91.3		
4	71.4		
Merchant signs present			
Yes	81.8		
No	73.9		
How the Merchant sells			
Over the Counter	77.8	**	*
Vending Machine	46.2		
Warning sign posted about the law			
Yes	82.5		
No	71.7		
Self-service tobacco display			
Yes	80.5		
No	76.8		
Special tobacco promotions			
Yes	75.5		
No	78.8		
Number of customers in line			
Nobody in line	74.9		
1 person in line	79.6		
2 people in line	71.4		
3 or more people in line	77.8		

* Indicates significance at $p \leq 0.05$
** Indicates significance at $p \leq 0.01$

There are several procedural limitations in the present study. Field Agents were instructed to state their true age, which probably lowered the sales rate in this study. Minors who actually intend to purchase cigarettes for personal use may lie about their age. The age of minors was restricted to just 15 and 16 years old and we only used females, so those studies that used a larger spread of minor

TABLE 2. Summary of Multivariate Multiple Logistic Regression Analysis for Variables Predicting Illegal Sales

Variables	%	estimate	odds ratio	95% CI	p value
	Sale Refused				
Clerk asked for age					
Yes	93.2	−4.219	.015	.012-.018	< .0001
No	72.2				
Clerk asked for ID					
Yes	97.5	−5.609	.004	.001-.027	< .0001
No	34.8				

ages and both genders probably are better able to assess the extent of these two characteristics on illegal sales. Field Agents were also instructed to state they did not have identification with them, and this probably also lowered the sales rate in this study. When Field Agents do not have an ID, this might make clerks more wary about selling cigarettes to a minor. In future studies, it is recommended that Field Agents present their IDs with their actual birthdate on it in response to a merchant request for age or ID. Employing this protocol would probably result in higher rates of illegal sales. It is important to recognize that some merchants probably would sell minors cigarettes when they present their own ID because they might not check the date on the ID to ascertain whether the minors were 18 or older (J. DiFranza, Personal Communication, November 30, 2000).

To restrict youth access to tobacco products, it is important for clerks to request identification from customers that appear to be minors and examine it to determine the age of the buyer. Our findings suggest that if a youth is asked for age or identification, it is less likely that clerks will sell cigarettes to minors. Although other factors have been implicated as affecting sales in other studies, and these factors also emerged in our univariate findings, multivariate methods indicate that the two important variables in influencing sales are merchant requests for age or ID. Future research should include these variables as important predictors of illegal sales.

REFERENCES

Arday, D.R., Klevens, R.M., Nelson, D.E., Huang, P., Giovino G.A., & Mowrey, P. (1997). Predictors of tobacco sales to minors. *Preventive Medicine, 26,* 8-13.

Centers for Disease Control. (1994). Attitudes toward smoking policies in eight states–United States, 1993. *Morbidity and Mortality Weekly Report, 43,* 786-789.

Clark, P.I., Natanblut, S.L., Schmitt, C.L., Wolters C., & Iachan, R. (2000). Factors associated with tobacco sales to minors. *Journal of the American Medical Association, 284*(6), 729-734.

DiFranza, J.R., Savageau, J.A., & Aisquith, B.F. (1996). Youth access to tobacco: The effects of age, gender, vending machine locks, and "It's the Law" programs. *American Journal of Public Health, 86*(2), 221-224.

Forster, J.L., Wolfson, M., Murray, D.M., Wagenaar, A.C., & Claxton, A.J. (1997). Perceived and measured availability of tobacco to youths in 14 Minnesota communities: The TPOP Study. *American Journal of Preventive Medicine, 13*(3), 167-175.

Gilpin, E.A., Choi, W.S., Berry, C., & Pierce, J.P. (1999). How many adolescents start smoking each day in the United States? *Journal of Adolescent Health, 25,* 248-255.

Hedeker, D., & Gibbons, R. D. (1996). MIXREG: A computer program for mixed-effects regression analysis with autocorrelated errors. *Computer Methods and Programs in Biomedicine, 49,* 229-252.

Jason, L.A., Berk, M., Schnopp-Wyatt, D.L., & Talbot, B. (1999). Effects of enforcement of youth access laws on smoking prevalence. *American Journal of Community Psychology, 27* (2), 143-160.

Jason, L.A., Biglan, A., & Katz, R. (1998). Implications of the tobacco settlement for the prevention of teenage smoking. *Childen's Services: Social Policy, Research, and Practice, 1,* 63-82.

Landrine, H., Klonoff, E.A., & Alcaraz, R. (1997). Asking age and identification may decrease minors' access to tobacco. *Preventive Medicine, 25,* 301-306.

O'Grady, B., Asbridge, M., & Abernathy, T. (1999). Analysis of factors related to illegal tobacco sales to young people in Ontario. *Tobacco Control, 8,* 301-305.

Rhodes, J.E., & Jason, L.A. (1988). *Preventing substance abuse among children and adolescents.* New York: Pergamon Press.

Wakefield, M., Terry, Y.M., Chaloupka, F., Barker, D.C., Slater, S., Clark, P.I., & Giovino, G.A. (2000). *Changes at the point-of-sale for tobacco following the 1999 tobacco billboard ban.* (Research Paper Series No. 4). Chicago, Illinois: University of Illinois at Chicago.

Examining Risks for Minors Participating in Tobacco Purchase Attempts

Peter Yun Ji
Steven B. Pokorny
Erin Blaszkowski
Leonard A. Jason
Olya Rabin-Belyaev

DePaul University

SUMMARY. This study aimed to provide empirical evidence to support previous research that participation in tobacco purchase attempt (TPA) procedures does not negatively impact minors' desire to initiate smoking habits or their willingness to discuss the dangers of smoking with peers and adults. Twenty-eight minors, who participated in TPAs, were compared to a group of eleven minors regarding whether or not they were smokers, whether or not they tried to get peers or adults to quit smoking, whether or not they tried to discuss with peers and adults about the dangers of smoking, and their perceptions of how easily it is to obtain tobacco products. Results demonstrated none of the minors in the TPA group initiated smoking, and there were not significant differences on most indicators regarding the frequency in which minors discussed the

Address correspondence to: Peter Yun Ji, PhD, Department of Psychology, DePaul University, 2219 N. Kenmore Avenue, Chicago, IL 60614.

The authors express appreciation for financial support provided by the Robert Wood Johnson Foundation and David Altman, the National Program Director, and Andrea Williams, the Deputy Director, of the Substance Abuse Policy Research Program.

[Haworth co-indexing entry note]: "Examining Risks for Minors Participating in Tobacco Purchase Attempts." Yun Ji, Peter et al. Co-published simultaneously in *Journal of Prevention & Intervention in the Community* (The Haworth Press, Inc.) Vol. 24, No. 1, 2002, pp. 77-85; and: *Preventing Youth Access to Tobacco* (ed: Leonard A. Jason, and Steven B. Pokorny) The Haworth Press, Inc., 2002, pp. 77-85. Single or multiple copies of this article are available for a fee from The Haworth Document Delivery Service [1-800-HAWORTH 9:00 a.m. - 5:00 p.m. (EST). E-mail address: getinfo@haworthpressinc.com].

dangers of smoking with peers and adults. Minors in both groups perceived that they could easily obtain tobacco products. The findings suggest that participation in TPAs does not adversely affect minors' intentions to smoke or their desire to initiate discussions about the dangers of smoking with peers and adults. *[Article copies available for a fee from The Haworth Document Delivery Service: 1-800-HAWORTH. E-mail address: <getinfo@haworthpressinc.com> Website: <http://www.HaworthPress.com>* © *2002 by The Haworth Press, Inc. All rights reserved.]*

KEYWORDS. Tobacco purchase, minors, risks, tobacco access

A growing prevention effort to keep minors from smoking tobacco is the restriction of the merchants' illegal sales of tobacco products. Nationwide, part of this effort involves enacting merchant tobacco control legislation, which penalizes merchants who sell tobacco to minors. Research has documented that these laws have dramatically reduced the sales of cigarettes to minors by tobacco merchant vendors (e.g., Feighery, Altman, & Shaffer, 1991; Forster, Komro, & Wolfson, 1996; Jason, Ji, Anes, & Birkhead, 1991).

The best method to test the effectiveness of these merchant tobacco control laws is to conduct merchant tobacco sales compliance checks (Radecki & Strohl, 1991; Jason, Berk, Schnopp-Wyatt, & Talbot, 1999). These compliance checks typically involve a minor, who is under the age of eighteen, as a field agent. The minor is sent into a store that sells tobacco products and attempts to purchase these products from the merchant vendor. If a merchant sells tobacco to the minor, then the merchant is considered to be in violation of the local ordinances that prohibit such sales. These checks are necessary because self-report measures or observational methods would likely be inaccurate or too cumbersome in assessing the rate of merchant tobacco sales to minors. Furthermore, these compliance checks must be done with a minor. If the compliance check were conducted with a person eighteen years of age or older, then the procedure would be invalid because technically the merchant did not sell tobacco to a minor.

There are several concerns about using minors to perform these compliance checks. One concern is that the compliance checks expose the minors to an illegal activity. In turn, this exposure could increase the likelihood that they too might begin illegally purchasing cigarettes on their own. A second concern is that if minors are exposed to the potential ease with which they could obtain cigarettes, they might attempt to start smoking. These are the concerns that most institutional review boards (IRB's) have regarding the use of minors in such operations. Indeed, a number of research efforts involving tobacco merchant compliance checks using minors have been rejected because of such concerns (Alcaraz, Klonoff, & Landrine, 1997). The aforementioned concerns are conceived as potential risks when using minors to perform merchant tobacco sales compliance checks. However, if these risks are being used to circumvent potential studies involving merchant tobacco compliance checks, then such concerns need to be empirically validated before they are considered as evidence to negate potentially useful studies.

One study has examined the impact of minors' participation in tobacco purchase attempts (TPA's) on the minors' likelihood that he or she will engage in smoking or illegal tobacco purchase attempts. Alcaraz et al. (1997) surveyed forty-eight minors who attended tobacco education workshops. Afterwards, thirty-six of these minors were randomly assigned to a TPA group. The remaining eleven minors were assigned to a control group that did not engage in TPA's attempt to purchase cigarettes. After surveying the minors two years later, the authors found that none of the minors initiated smoking habits. Furthermore, some of the minors in the TPA group were influential in helping their parents quit smoking or asking friends not to smoke. Thus, the minors' participation in the TPA's did not increase the likelihood of commencing smoking habits. In fact, the authors felt that having minors involved in TPA's would actually be an effective prevention effort to help keep minors and their peers from using tobacco.

The purpose of the present study was meant to examine the issues explored in Alacraz et al. (1997). The present study hypothesized that minors who engage in TPA's will not engage in future tobacco use. This study also investigated how participating in TPA's would impact minors' impression of their ability to obtain tobacco from merchants.

METHOD

Participants

Field Agents. In each town, only non-smoking female youth aged 15 or 16 were recruited as field agents for this project. Informed, active consent was necessary from both the youth and one of their parents/legal guardians in order for the youth to participate in the Tobacco Purchase Attempts. The liaison police officer was asked to confirm that participating youth actually looked 15 or 16 years old by obtaining two Visual Age Assessment Ratings for each youth. Caucasian and Non-White females participated as field agents in the Tobacco Purchase Attempts across the communities. Youth were paid $5 per hour.

Tobacco Purchase Attempt Protocol. A standard protocol was utilized for completing the Tobacco Purchase Attempts (TPA) (Jason, Engstrom, Pokorny, Tegart, & Curie, 2000). When asked for their age during any type of Tobacco Purchase Attempt, Field Agents responded by stating their true age. When asked for identification during any type of Tobacco Purchase Attempt, Field Agents stated, "I'm sorry, I don't have my ID with me."

Demographic Information. Twenty-eight minors, who participated in TPA's, consented to be surveyed and were considered the TPA group. A total of eleven minors comprised the comparison group, of which eight minors were recruited at a local high school. Three minors were referred for the comparison group by the minors who participated in the TPA's.

The minors in both groups were female. The mean age of the participant was 15.95 (SD = .72, range = 15-17). Of the females, 18 (46.2%) were Sophomores, 19 (48.7%) were Juniors, and 2 were Seniors (5.1%) in high school. Their ethnic classification was 31 (79.5%) Caucasian, 2 (5.1%) Black, 4 (10.3%) Hispanic, and 2 (5.1%) Asian.

T-tests were conducted and indicated that there was a significant difference in the mean ages of the minors between the TPA group and the comparison group (t [36] = 2.32, $p < .05$). Specifically, the minors in the TPA group were approximately a half year older than those in the Comparison group (TPA mean age = 16.18, SD = .72 vs. Comparison group mean age = 15.60, SD = .52).

Chi-square tests were conducted and indicated that there was a significant difference in the number of Caucasian and Non-Caucasian minors in the TPA and Comparison groups (χ^2 (1) = 10.88, $p < .01$). In the TPA group, 26 (92.9%) were Caucasian, 2 (7.1%) were Non-Caucasians, whereas in the comparison group, 5 (45.5%) were Caucasians and 6 (54.5%) were Non-Caucasians.

Materials

The survey consisted of eight questions. The minors were asked: (a) if they were currently a cigarette smoker, (b) how easy would it be for them to get tobacco products if they wanted to, (c) during the last school year, how frequently did they talk to friends or peers about the dangers of smoking, (d) have they ever tried to get a friend or peer to quit smoking?, (e) during the last school year, how many friends or peers have you tried to get to quit smoking, (f) during the last school year, how frequently would you say that they talked to an adult about the dangers of smoking, and (g) during the last school year, how many adults have you tried to get to quit smoking? Depending on the nature of the questions, minors responded with either a yes or no response or on a likert scale response.

Procedure

The Youth Tobacco Access Project staff served as the interviewers for this study. Minors in both groups were contacted via telephone interviews. Each interview lasted between fifteen and twenty minutes. The initial interview was conducted within one month of the minors' participation in the TPA's. The follow-up interview occurred six months later. All of the minors who participated in the first round of interviews participated in the six-month follow-up interview.

RESULTS

There were no significant differences between the TPA group and the comparison group regarding the number of minors who considered themselves a current smoker at the initial and follow-up interview [initial interview (χ^2 (3, N = 39) = .47), follow-up interview (χ^2 (3, N = 39) = 2.97)]. At the follow-up interview, none of the 28 TPA field agents began smoking, but one of the minors in the comparison group began smoking.

There were no significant differences between the TPA group and the comparison group regarding how easy the minors felt they could obtain tobacco products at either the initial or follow-up interview: Within-Subjects $F(1,37)$ = .79; Interaction $F(1,37)$ = .79; Between-Subjects $F(1,37)$ = .04. Minors in both groups felt it was easy to obtain tobacco products.

There were no significant differences over time for either the TPA group and the comparison group in the frequency the minors talked to their friends or peers about dangers of smoking: Within-Subjects $F(1, 36)$ = .01; Interaction $F(1,36)$ = .34. However, there was an overall significant difference between the TPA group and the comparison group: Between-Subjects F(1, 36) = 6.91, $p < .05$. Minors in the control group were more likely to talk to their friends or peers about the dangers of smoking than minors in the TPA group.

There were no significant differences between the TPA group and the comparison group regarding whether or not the minors had ever tried to get a friend or peer to quit smoking at the initial and follow-up interview [initial interview (χ^2 (1, N = 39) = 1.00), follow-up interview (χ^2 (1, N = 39) = .02)]. At the follow-up interview, in the TPA group, 21 (75%) minors indicated they had tried to get a peer to quit smoking, while in the comparison group, 8 (72.7%) minors indicated they had tried to get a peer to quit smoking.

There were no significant differences between the TPA group and the comparison group regarding how many friends or peers have they tried to get to quit smoking during the last school year at the initial and follow-up interview: Within-Subjects F(1,36) = 3.64; Interaction F (1,36) = .82; Between-Subjects F(1,36) = .37. Minors in both groups reported trying to get at least two friends or peers to quit smoking.

There were no significant differences between the TPA group and the comparison group regarding how frequently they talked to an adult about the dangers of smoking at the initial and follow-up interview: Within-Subjects F(1,36) = .02; Interaction F(1,36) = .11; Between-Subjects F(1,36) = 1.10. Minors in both groups reported talking to an adult about smoking an average of once per month.

There were no significant differences between the TPA group and the comparison group regarding whether or not the minors had ever tried to get an adult at the initial and follow-up interview [initial interview (χ^2 (1, N = 38) = .30), follow-up interview (χ^2 (1, N = 39) = .07)]. At the follow-up interview, in the TPA group, 14 (50%) minors indicated they had tried to get a peer to quit smoking, while in the comparison group, 6 (54.5%) minors indicated they had tried to get a peer to quit smoking.

There were no significant differences between the TPA group and the comparison group regarding how many adults the minors tried to get to quit smoking during the past school year at the initial and follow-up interview: Within-Subjects F (1,36) = .83; Interaction F (1,36) = .83; Between-Subjects F (1,36) = .23. Minors in both groups reported trying to get at least one adult to quit smoking.

DISCUSSION

Our results indicate there were no negative effects for minors who participated in TPAs. All of the minors in the TPA group did not consider themselves to be a current smoker at the initial and six-month follow-up, while one minor in the comparison group did report being a smoker at the six-month follow-up. The results are consistent with Alcaraz et al. (1997)'s findings that minors who participate in TPAs are no more likely than their peers who did not participate in TPA's to begin cigarette smoking.

Minors in both groups indicated they felt it was easy to purchase tobacco products. This result could reflect what research on illegal tobacco sales to minors has already confirmed: without stringent merchant tobacco sales control legislation, minors can easily obtain cigarettes from merchants. The finding that minors in the TPA group were just as likely as minors in the comparison group to perceive that they could easily obtain tobacco products is not surprising. After minors participated in TPAs in a community where there are no active merchant tobacco control laws, they would realize that merchants would readily sell tobacco products to minors. However, as Alcaraz et al. (1997) demonstrated, minors usually expressed disgust that they could easily obtain tobacco products, which led to stronger anti-tobacco use among themselves and their peers. Thus, although minors, by participating in TPAs, would perceive they could easily obtain tobacco products via merchants, it is also quite likely they would be displeased at the lack of control over merchants' illegal tobacco sales to minors.

It appears that participating in TPAs did not adversely affect minors' desire to talk with their friends or adults about the dangers of smoking or their desire to get their peers or adults to quit smoking. However, minors in the comparison group more frequently talked to friends or peers about the dangers of smoking than minors in the TPA group. We expected that minors in the TPA group would be more likely than minors in the comparison group to talk with their friends or peers about the dangers of smoking, so this result was contrary to what was expected. However, the result does indicate that minors who participated in TPAs did engage in discussing the dangers of smoking with their friends and peers. These results are consistent with Alcaraz et al. (1997), in which there were no differences between minors who participated in TPAs and a control group of minors regarding the presence or absence of discussing the issue of smoking with their friends.

One limitation of the study is its sample size. A total of thirty-five minors participated and less than half of the minors were assigned to the comparison group. Thus, some of the observed effects could be due to the small sample size. Future research should attempt to replicate these results with a larger and more balanced sample size between experimental and control groups. Second, the minors who participated in this study were all girls and most were Caucasian. Thus, future research could examine if these effects are consistent for both boys and girls and for other ethnic groups as well. Third, there were some differences in the ages and the ethnic classification between the TPA group and the comparison group. It is unknown how the demographic differences between the two groups might have impacted the results, but future research could examine these possibilities. Fourth, no pre-test was given before the minors participated in the TPAs so comparisons regarding if the TPA experienced had an effect on minors' perceptions of tobacco use and illegal sales cannot be ascertained. It would be worthwhile to determine if participation in TPAs leads to a significant positive impact on minors' desires to advocate for the cessation of smoking among their peers or adults and to lobby for the restriction of merchant tobacco sales to minors.

Overall, the findings suggest that minors who participate in TPAs are likely not to experience any negative effects, are no more at risk in engaging in smoking habits, and are likely to discuss the dangers of smoking with their friends and adults. The findings are similar to previous findings, which indicate that TPAs pose minimal risks to minors. Thus, concerns about whether or not minors would engage in tobacco use or other negative effects as a result of their participation in TPAs remains unfounded. Based on the findings to date, TPAs can still be used as an effective method to test the effectiveness of merchant tobacco sales control legislation and minors who participate in TPAs may actually initiate positive discussions among peers and adults about the dangers of smoking.

REFERENCES

Alcaraz, R., Klonoff, E. A., & Landrine, H. (1997). The effects on children of participating in studies of minors' access to tobacco. *Preventive Medicine, 26,* 236-240.
Feighery, M. S., Altman, D. G., & Shaffer, M. A. (1991). The effects of combining education and enforcement to reduce tobacco sales to minors. *Journal of the American Medical Association, 266,* 3168-3171.

Forster, J.L., Komro, K. A., & Wolfson, M. (1996). Survey of city ordinances and local enforcement regarding commercial availability of tobacco to minors in Minnesota, United States. *Tobacco Control, 5*, 46-51.

Jason, L. A., Berk, M., Schnopp-Wyatt, D. L., & Talbot, B. (1999). Effects of enforcement of youth access laws on smoking prevalence. *American Journal of Community Psychology, 27*(2), 143-160.

Jason, L.A., Engstrom, M. D., Pokorny, S.B., Tegart, G., & Curie, C.J. (2000). Putting the community back into prevention: Think locally, act globally. *The Journal of Primary Prevention, 21*, 25-29.

Jason, L. A., Ji, P. Y., Anes, M., & Birkhead, S. H. (1991). Active enforcement of cigarette control laws in the prevention of cigarette sales to minors. *Journal of American Medical Association, 266*(22), 3159-3161.

Radecki, T. E., & Strohl, J. (1991). Survey of underage youth and alcohol purchase habits in 17 Midwest and Eastern states. *Drug Free Youth News, 1*, 1-8.

A Response to the Critiques
of Tobacco Sales
and Tobacco Possession Laws

Leonard A. Jason
Steven B. Pokorny

DePaul University

Michael E. Schoeny

University of Illinois at Chicago

SUMMARY. Several researchers within the anti-smoking community have recently claimed that youth access tobacco programs are ineffective and drain limited resources. They make these claims because they feel that youth access programs do not affect teen smoking prevalence. Others have argued that anti-smoking interventions should not fine minors for possession of tobacco. In this last article, we provide a response to these arguments. *[Article copies available for a fee from The Haworth Document Delivery Service: 1-800-HAWORTH. E-mail address: <getinfo@haworthpressinc.com> Website: <http://www.HaworthPress.com> © 2002 by The Haworth Press, Inc. All rights reserved.]*

Address correspondence to: Leonard A. Jason, PhD, DePaul University, Center for Community Research, 990 West Fullerton Avenue, Chicago, IL 60614.

The authors express appreciation for financial support provided by the Robert Wood Johnson Foundation and David Altman, the National Program Director, and Andrea Williams, the Deputy Director, of the Substance Abuse Policy Research Program.

[Haworth co-indexing entry note]: "A Response to the Critiques of Tobacco Sales and Tobacco Possession Laws." Jason, Leonard A., Steven B. Pokorny, and Michael E. Schoeny. Co-published simultaneously in *Journal of Prevention & Intervention in the Community* (The Haworth Press, Inc.) Vol. 24, No. 1, 2002, pp. 87-95; and: *Preventing Youth Access to Tobacco* (ed: Leonard A. Jason, and Steven B. Pokorny) The Haworth Press, Inc., 2002, pp. 87-95. Single or multiple copies of this article are available for a fee from The Haworth Document Delivery Service [1-800-HAWORTH 9:00 a.m. - 5:00 p.m. (EST). E-mail address: getinfo@haworthpressinc.com].

KEYWORDS. Youth access tobacco programs, measurement, prevention, public health

In a recent editorial, Ling, Landman and Glantz (2002) argue that youth access tobacco programs are ineffective and drain limited resources. They argue that these programs do not affect teen smoking prevalence (Fichtenberg & Glantz, 2002) because as fewer merchants sell tobacco to minors, teens will use social sources to obtain tobacco. The authors further claim that these programs help build coalitions for the tobacco industry. Wakefield and Giovino (2002), on the other hand, argue that teen penalties for tobacco possession may divert public efforts from more effective anti-smoking strategies, and these policies are unlikely to reduce youth smoking at the population level. In this article, we provide a response to these arguments.

The tobacco industry's programs in the early to mid 1990s that are cited in Ling et al.'s (2002) editorial were primarily focused on educational campaigns, which did not include merchant fines for selling to minors. The Tobacco Industry was forced to accept programs that fined merchants rather than ineffective educational programs, and now Ling et al. (2002) argue for eliminating these monitoring and fining programs that have been embraced by communities throughout the US and other countries. The likely result of reversing this fining policy would be that the majority of merchants would once again sell minors tobacco. Teens would receive mixed messages about tobacco use, as they would be urged not to start smoking in schools and at the same time being provided easy access to this dangerous drug by adult role models who manage businesses in the community.

One problem with previous studies that have investigated the relation of Retail Tobacco Availability (RTA) to youth tobacco use is that they measured this factor as the number of retailers who illegally sold out of the number of tobacco retailers assessed (Altman et al., 1999; Forster et al., 1998; Jason et al., 1991; Rigotti et al., 1997). This approach does not account for the relative density of tobacco retailers in each community, which may affect the likelihood that a youth will encounter a retailer who is not compliant with the tobacco sales law. In contrast, a more appropriate measure of risk exposure would reflect the number of retailers who illegally sold tobacco as a function of the youth population (i.e., youth between the ages of 10 and 17) within each community.

A recent study that assessed the rate of illegal retail tobacco sales to minors illustrates some important differences in measures of youth access to tobacco (Pokorny, Jason, & Schoeny, in press). Table 1 provides information from 11 communities and their groupings sorted by different measures of RTA (i.e., population adjusted). As shown in Table 1, there are important differences between the traditional measure of RTA (i.e., percent of retailers who sold) and a new risk index for the measurement of RTA (i.e., retailers who sold per 1000 youth). For example, data from Towns 6 and 7 suggests some important inconsistencies. Using the traditional measure of RTA, Town 7 has only 17% of retailers selling tobacco, and thus it would be considered as in compliance with the Synar amendment, which stipulates that states need to keep merchant illegal sales rates of tobacco to minors under 20% (Jacobson, Wasserman & Anderson, 1997). In contrast, Town 6 has more than twice the rate of illegal tobacco sales to minors than Town 7 using the traditional measure of RTA (36%), and thus would be considered as having a rather high level of tobacco accessible to children. However, using the new risk index of RTA, the number of retailers who sold per 1000 youth in Town 6 is actually lower than Town 7. The index of risk exposure that includes retailers who sell per 1000 may provide a more sensitive assessment than that used by previous studies (Pokorny et al., in press).

In the Pokorny et al. (in press) mentioned above, individual, social, and environmental influences on smoking initiation and continued smoking

TABLE 1. Characteristics of Communities (N = 11)

Town	Youth Population	Number of Retailers	Number of Retailers Who Sold	Percent of Retailers Who Sold	Number of Retailers Who Sold per 1000 Youth
1	1,474	17	1	.06	.7
2	10,612	63	8	.13	.7
3	1,773	21	3	.14	1.7
4	925	12	2	.17	2.2
5	1,981	19	5	.26	2.5
6	9,271	67	24	.36	2.6
7	1,389	23	4	.17	2.9
8	1,789	25	6	.24	3.3
9	4,188	35	17	.49	4.1
10	811	17	4	.24	4.9
11	1,288	17	7	.41	5.4

among sixth, seventh, and eighth grade students was examined using this new RTA index. Greater retail tobacco availability was positively associated with smoking initiation but not continued cigarette use. Restrictions in retail tobacco availability may prevent youth from initiating smoking, but may have less impact on those addicted to tobacco. The Fichtenberg and Glanz (2002) meta-analysis only examined current smoking rather than smoking initiation.

Typically, youth who conduct retail tobacco access assessments are not permitted to lie about their age, use an ID card, dress to appear older, purchase other items, or engage the clerk in irrelevant friendly conversation. It is with these types of procedures that low rates of illegal tobacco sales have been found. This research protocol may be more similar to methods used by youth who are less experienced at purchasing cigarettes. However, when youth who are experienced at purchasing tobacco are allowed to use their usual purchase methods (e.g., appear as they want, purchase other items, lie about their age, present a valid ID, and engage the clerk in conversation), they are six times more likely to obtain cigarettes from clerks than youth who use methods required by standard assessment protocol (DiFranza, Savageau, & Bouchard, 2001). In other words, compliance check procedures used in programs to restrict retail tobacco availability may be successful in limiting relatively inexperienced smokers from purchasing cigarettes, but these programs to limit youth access to tobacco might be less successful for addicted smokers, who are able to use more sophisticated methods to purchase cigarettes. The fact that young smokers are beginning to shift to social sources for tobacco (Jones, Sharp, Husten, & Crossett, 2002) suggests that for some youth smokers, the barriers to purchasing retail tobacco are strengthening. Rather than reducing these obstacles to youth access to tobacco, it might be more appropriate to assess the effects of even tougher barriers to retail and social sources of tobacco.

Several studies have found that tobacco-control policies, which might be influencing norms that impact retail and social sources, have reduced prevalence of youth smoking. A longitudinal, statewide study in Massachusetts found that youths living in communities with local tobacco sales laws were less likely to progress to established smoking over a four-year period than were youths living in communities without such laws (Siegel, Biener, & Rigotti, 1999). In addition, a national study of state youth tobacco control policies found that youths living in states with more comprehensive policies had significantly lower rates of smoking than did youths living in states without such policies (Luke, Stamatakis, & Brownson, 2000).

The effectiveness of youth possession laws have been challenged on a theoretical basis because youth smoking has a low likelihood of detection, youth may actively avoid detection, and there is an impersonal relationship between punisher and recipient (Wakefield & Giovino, 2002). Clearly, youth possession laws can be implemented poorly, but the same can be said for school-based tobacco prevention programs and media-based programs. The key issue is whether when implemented appropriately, do youth possession laws avoid the problems mentioned by Wakefield and Giovino (2002), and whether such programs have the potential to reduce youth smoking.

In Woodridge, Illinois, Officer Talbot first introduced into his community a law that included a provision that prohibited the possession and use of tobacco by minors. Violations of this provision were considered civil rather than criminal offenses that result in a ticket carrying a $25 fine and parental notification of the incident. The possession provision was created to send a clear message that youth could not purchase or use tobacco in the community. Officer Talbot wanted this provision because he often observed youth congregating and smoking in front of the entrance to youth events (e.g., school dances), and he was powerless to stop them from modeling this negative behavior in front of other impressionable youth. He also felt that the presence of these groups contributed to the misperception that the majority of youth smoked and suggested that it was an acceptable community norm for youth to use tobacco. Officer Talbot wanted a law that would give him the authority to intervene and stop groups of youth using tobacco at these events because he believed that his actions could help to change community norms regarding youth tobacco use. These types of laws have strong community support, from both the parents and youth; the consequences are delivered by police who only enforce this law when youth are already engaged in another illegal activity (just as police give out seat belt citations only after a driver is caught speeding); and the law aims at creating changes in norms within the community rather than serving as a deterrent to a particular individual.

Wakefield and Giovino (2002) claim that it is unlikely that these minor possession laws will exert a general deterrent effect because many parents and teens do not know about these laws and that the rates of enforcement compared to the rates of violations are extremely small. Clearly, it is important to adequately publicize these types of laws when they are implemented, and when such efforts occur, most youngsters do become aware of the laws. For example, in the Robert Wood Johnson study mentioned in the first chapter (Jason, Pokorny, & Schoeny,

2002), the vast majority of the youth were aware of the possession law (e.g., 74% of the eighth graders were aware of this law, L. Jason, Personal Communication, July 17, 2002). In addition, at an eight-year follow-up, data from Woodridge, IL indicated that only 4.5% had been caught or disciplined for smoking (Jason, Katz et al., 1999) and this suggests that enforcements only occur for a small minority of the smokers, and what is important is for the teens to know that there is the possibility of there being an enforcement, not necessarily that all youngsters who smoke will be ticketed. In fact, we found both in Woodridge and in the Robert Wood Johnson Foundation-supported study that when tickets were given out, over time the police had more difficulties finding youth who were smoking in public, and as a consequence, the number of fines in these communities decreased over time.

Clearly, we feel it is inappropriate for communities to only cite minors for tobacco possession and not attempt to reduce merchant illegal tobacco sales. We believe that it is inappropriate to devote more resources and time to prosecuting minors for possession of tobacco than for prosecuting retailers for violation of sales to minors laws, and unfortunately, this has occurred in some communities (Forster, Komro, & Wolfson, 1996). The work our research team has engaged in over the past decade has always first focused on reducing illegal merchant tobacco sales, and then focusing on the issue of teen penalties for possession of tobacco. Our group feels strongly that to punish youth for possession of alcohol and other illicit drugs, but to allow them to use tobacco, sends a mixed message that indicates that tobacco is less dangerous than alcohol or other drugs, and this is damaging to our efforts to bring about new anti-smoking norms. The idea has also been forwarded that these possession laws divert resources from other anti-smoking activities, and even help tobacco companies and retailers gather support for more regressive policies. When states have these types of laws that pre-empt local laws that could be more comprehensive, we feel that these practices need to be challenged. We support local laws because they can be both stronger and better enforced. Our experience in Illinois has suggested that at the local level, when communities are empowered to see changes in illegal sales rates of tobacco or fewer minors smoking in public, this leads them not only to feel successful for their efforts but also to become even more confident in initiating other anti-smoking efforts. This is in stark contrast with what often occurs when community coalitions set unclear objectives that are difficult to evaluate, and therefore, community members are unclear about the success of their anti-smoking campaigns.

Several investigators have found that enforced school polices are associated with reduced smoking by youth (Pinilla et al., 2002; Wakefield et al., 2000), and youth possession laws could be coordinated to strengthen enforcement of these policies. In addition, others have found that youth possession laws might even influence youth to quit smoking. In Minnesota, Lazovitch et al. (2001) found 18.9% quit smoking after they had paid a fine ($50 for the first offense and $75 for the second offense) for tobacco possession whereas 15.5% quit after attending a 2 and a half hour tobacco education class and a $25 fine; given the low rates of quitting among teen quitting programs, these rates are rather respectable. Additional supportive data comes from Florida, where Langer and Wahrheit (2000) studied youth who were cited for possession violations and where the youth and their parents had to appear in court and watch a video on the health effects of smoking, and then were fined, provided community service or mandated to attend a tobacco education class. At a two-month follow-up, 28% claimed to have not used tobacco. Finally, also in Florida, Livingood et al. (2001) compared teen smoking in two counties with high rates of minor possession enforcement and two counties with low levels, and they found that the high enforcement communities were significantly associated with reduced likelihood of currently smoking.

Jason, Berk et al. (1999) found that high school youths who lived in communities with regular enforcement of youth access and possession policies had significantly lower rates of smoking compared to youths who lived in communities without such enforcement. The study by Jason, Pokorny and Schoeny (2002), described in the first article in this volume, had findings that were supportive of these types of laws. There has been considerable attention focused on whether youth in towns that have fines for possession of tobacco develop negative attitudes toward these policies. In the Jason et al. (2002) study findings indicated that youth in the P (teen fine plus merchant sale law enforcement condition) in comparison to youth in the NP (just merchant sale condition) had generally fewer negative attitudes over time toward these fining policies. When asked if minors should be fined for possessing or using tobacco, the percent who disagreed or strongly disagreed with these policies increased over the three-year study for white P youth from 12.1% to 16.19% and for white NP youth from 15.7% to 31.3%; for non-white P youth, from 14.5% to 22.8% and for non-white NP youth, from 20.6% to 35.8%.

In Ling et al.'s (2002) editorial, we are told to abandon youth access programs and instead focus on other public health measures such as taxes, media campaigns and smoke-free workplaces and homes. However, these public health initiatives are not free of unintended side effects, as raising taxes can lead to more theft or even black market smuggling, media campaigns are often overwhelmed by counter advertising efforts, and smoke-free work settings can lead to people congregating at building entrances modeling this negative behavior. We believe that it is too early to eliminate youth access programs and youth possession laws, as they represent one of the more popular vehicles for galvanizing public support for anti-smoking activities and establishing social norms against youth tobacco use. Moreover, given the methodological limitations of the current research (DiFranza, 2002), future research with more rigorous and controlled designs might indicate that such interventions, particularly those that change social norms, might even have a role in reducing smoking initiation and prevalence rates.

REFERENCES

Altman, D.G., Wheelis, A.Y., McFarlane, M., Hye-ryeon, L., & Fortmann, S.P. (1999). The relationship between tobacco access and use among adolescents: A four community study. *Social Science and Medicine, 48,* 759-775.

DiFranza, J.R. (2002). It is time to abandon bad science. *Tobacco Control* [Electronic Letter to the Editor, May 13, 2002]

DiFranza, J.R., Savageau, J.A., & Bouchard, J. (2001). Is the standard compliance check protocol a valid measure of the accessibility of tobacco to underage smokers? *Tobacco Control, 10,* 227-232.

Fichtenberg, C.M., & Glantz, S.A. (2002). Youth access interventions do not affect youth smoking. *Pediatrics,* 109, 1087-1091.

Forster, J. L., Komro, K. A., & Wolfson, M. (1996). Survey of city ordinances and local enforcement regarding commercial availability of tobacco to minors in Minnesota, United States. *Tobacco Control, 5,* 46-51.

Forster, J.L., Murray, D.M., Wolfson, M., Blaine, T.M., Wagenaar, A.C., & Hennrikus, D.J. (1998). The effects of community policies to reduce youth access to tobacco. *American Journal of Public Health, 88* (8), 1193-1198.

Jacobson, P.D., Wassermen, J., & Anderson, J.R. (1997). Historical overview of tobacco legislation. *Journal of Social Issues, 53,* 75-95.

Jason, L.A., Berk, M., Schnopp-Wyatt, D.L., & Talbot, B. (1999). Effects of enforcement of youth access laws on smoking prevalence. *American Journal of Community Psychology, 27* (2), 143-160.

Jason, L.A., Ji, P.Y., Anes, M.D., & Birkhead, S.H. (1991). Active enforcement of cigarette control laws in the prevention of cigarette sales to minors. *The Journal of the American Medical Association, 266* (22), 3159-3161.

Jason, L.A., Katz, R., Vavra, J., & Schnopp-Wyatt, D.L. (1999). Long term follow-up of youth access to tobacco laws' impact on smoking prevalence. *Journal of Human Behavior in the Social Environment, 2,* 1-13.

Jason, L.A., Pokorny, S.B., & Schoeny, M.E. (2002, August). Evaluating the effects of enforcements and fines on youth smoking. Paper presented at the annual meeting of the American Psychological Association, Chicago, IL.

Jones, S.E., Sharp, D.J., Husten, C.G., & Crosett, L.S. (2002). Cigarette acquisition and proof of age among US high school students who smoke. *Tobacco Control, 11,* 20-25.

Langer, L.M., & Warheit, G.J. (2000). Teen tobacco court: A determination of the short-term outcomes of judicial processes with teens engaging in tobacco possession. *Adolescent Family Health, 1,* 5-10.

Lazovich, D., Ford, J., Forster, J., & Riley, B. (2001). A pilot study to evaluate a tobacco diversion program. *American Journal of Public Health, 91,* 1790-1791.

Ling, P.M., Landman, A., & Glantz, S.A. (2002). Is it time to abandon youth access tobacco programmes? *Tobacco Control, 11,* 3-6.

Livingood, W.C., Woodhouse, C.D., Sayre, J.J., & Wludka, P. (2001). Impact study of tobacco possession law enforcement in Florida. *Health Education Behavior, 28,* 733-748.

Luke, D.A., Stamatakis, K.A., & Brownson, R.C. (2000). State youth-access tobacco control policies and youth smoking behavior in the United States. *American Journal of Preventive Medicine, 19,* 180-187.

Pinilla, J., Gonzalez, B., Barber, P., & Santana, Y. (2002). Smoking in young adolescents: An approach with multilevel discrete choice models. *Journal of Epidemiology and Community Health, 56,* 227-232.

Pokorny, S.B., Jason, L.A, & Schoeny, M.E. (in press). Effects of retail tobacco availability on initiation and continued cigarette smoking. *Journal of Clinical Child and Adolescent Psychology.*

Rigotti, N. A., DiFranza, J. R., Chang, Y., Tisdale, T., Kemp, B., & Singer, D. E. (1997). The effects of enforcing tobacco-sales laws on adolescents' access to tobacco and smoking behavior. *The New England Journal of Medicine, 337* (15), 1044-1051.

Siegel, M., Biener, L., & Rigotti, N.A. (1999). The effect of local tobacco sales laws on adolescent smoking initiation. *Preventive Medicine, 29,* 334-342.

Wakefield, M.A., Chaloupka, F.J., Kaufman, N.J., Orleans, C.T., Barker, D.C., & Ruel, E.E. (2000). Effect of restrictions on smoking at home, at school, and in public places on teenage smoking: Cross-sectional study. *British Medical Journal, 321,* 333-337.

Wakefield, M., & Giovino, G. (2002, July). Teen penalties for tobacco possession, use and purchase: Evidence and issues. Paper presented at the Innovations in Youth Tobacco Control Conference, Sante Fe, New Mexico.

Index

Access prevention
  CDC (Centers for Disease Control)
    and, 2
  HHS (U. S. Dept. of Health and
    Human Services) and, 4-5
  influence factors and, 63-76. *See
    also* Influence factors
  introduction to
    background data about, 1-3
    community program
      effectiveness, 10-11
    easy *vs.* restricted access, 3-7
    future perspectives of, 11
    reference and research literature
      about, 11-13
    research about, 8-10
    solutions for, 4-5
  law quality measures, 15-27. *See
    also* Law quality measures
  Robert Wood Johnson Foundation
    and, 8-10
  sales and possession laws, 87-95.
    See also Sales and possession
    laws
  SAMHSA (Substance Abuse and
    Mental Health Services
    Administration) regulations
    and, 4-5
  school-based programs, 47-61. *See
    also* School-based prevention
    programs
  stage theory-multi-community
    intervention applications and,
    29-46. *See also* Stage
    theory-multi-community
    intervention applications
  Synar Amendment and, 5

TPA (tobacco purchase attempt)
    procedures and, 77-85. *See
    also* TPA (tobacco purchase
    attempt) procedures
Act-L (Assessment of the
    Comprehensiveness of
    Tobacco Laws) Scale, 20-22
Advocacy, media, 24
Age characteristics, 65-66
American Legacy Foundation, 48-49
Assessment of the Comprehensiveness
    of Youth Tobacco Control
    Laws, 20-22,26-27

Blaszkowski, E., 77-85
Buyer characteristics, 64-75

CDC (Centers for Disease Control),
    2,48-59,64-65
Change, stages of, 33-36
Clerk characteristics and behaviors,
    65-66,70-75
Community readiness models, 29-46
Compliance checks, sales, 78-79
Comprehensive approaches, 17-18
Conceptual heuristics, 37-38
CSAP (Center for Substance Abuse
    Prevention), 49-55
Curie, C. J.
  access prevention, research about,
    1-13
  influence factors, research about,
    63-76
  school-based prevention programs,
    research about, 47-61